COPING with your GROWN CHILDREN

COPING

with your

GROWN

CHILDREN

by

Edwin L. Klingelhofer

Humana Press • Clifton, New Jersey

© Copyright 1989 by The Humana Press Inc.
Crescent Manor
PO Box 2148
Clifton, NJ 07015

Library of Congress Cataloging-in-Publication Data

Klingelhofer, E. L. (Ed. L.)
  Coping with your grown children.

  Includes index.
  1. Adult children—United States—Family relationships.
  2. Adult children—United States—Psychology. I. Title.
HQ799.97.U5K55   1989   646.7'8   88-13734
ISBN 0-89603-159-4

Dedication

This is for Jean
And our kids
And our kids' kids

Preface

Millions of today's middle-aged parents are encountering a seeming plague of problems with their grown children. Problems of cohabitation—homosexuality—drug and alcohol abuse—failure to live up to potential—failure to leave home at all—these are each high among the predicaments in their children's lives that all too many middle-aged parents today can neither comprehend nor successfully manage.

Coping with Your Grown Children identifies many of the often complex roots and expressions of these new troubles and then moves on to trace some of the recent, explosive social changes that have brought them about.

It spotlights the almost irresistible tendency for parents to assume blame for the difficulties, the shortcomings, and the failures of their children. It reminds these parents that forces outside the home—forces quite often beyond the knowledge or control of the parents—influence their children mightily.

It shows that family conflicts may seriously imperil the physical and psychological well-being of the very many troubled middle-aged parents for whom this book has been written.

And it introduces the frequently hurt and perplexed parent to effective and constructive ways of approaching and resolving these problems.

Edwin L. Klingelhofer

Acknowledgments

This book owes much to many:
- The friends and clients—middle-aged parents—who pointed up the need for and suggested much of the book's direction and content
- The students who zealously accepted the invitation to criticize, comment and correct
- The colleagues who read and improved the manuscript in its several drafts—especially Geeta Dardick, Ernie Isaacs, Walter Schenkel
- Tom Lanigan who made it ever so better than it was
- And, the people whose thoughts provide chapter preambles. Among them several bumper sticker aphorists, Dorothy Clark, Sir William Drummond, Frederick the Great, Sigmund Freud, Proverbs XX, William Shakespeare, Pat Swanson, and Rabindrinath Tagore.

Thanks are also owed to
- Dear Abby: for permission to reprint the material appearing on page 157; Copyright 1987 Universal Press Syndicate Reprinted with permission. All rights reserved.
- Ann Landers, and the *Los Angeles Times* Syndicate, and the *Sacramento Union* for permission to reprint the material appearing on page 57
- Thomas McGuane and Random House Inc., for permission to reprint, from Mr. McGuane's *Something to be Desired*, 1984, page 22, the material appearing on page 103.

E.L.K.

Contents

PART ONE

THE PROBLEMS WITH ADULT CHILDREN

PART TWO

DEFINING AND LOCATING YOUR PROBLEM

PART THREE

SHARED PROBLEMS
OF PARENTS AND ADULT CHILDREN

CHAPTER 13
Lifestyles and Meaningful Relationships

CHAPTER 14
Gay or Lesbian Children

CHAPTER 15
Cult Memberships

CHAPTER 16
Abuse of Substances

CHAPTER 17
The Ungrateful Child

PART FIVE

COPING STRATEGIES

CHAPTER 18
How to Develop a Rational Solution for Your
Parent–Child Problem: *Building a Decision-Tree*

CHAPTER 19
An Exercise in Decision-Making

CHAPTER 20
Finding the Right Kind of Help

PART ONE

The Problems
with Adult Children

Millions of today's middle-aged parents are encountering a seeming plague of problems with their grown children. Problems of cohabitation—homosexuality—drug and alcohol abuse—failure to live up to potential—failure to leave home at all—these are each high among the predicaments in their children's lives that all too many middle-aged parents today can neither comprehend nor successfully manage.

This first part of *Coping with Your Grown Children* identifies many of the often complex roots and expressions of these new troubles and then moves on to trace some of the recent, explosive social changes that have brought them about.

It spotlights the almost irresistible tendency for parents to assume blame for the difficulties, the shortcomings, and the failures of their children. It reminds these parents that forces outside the home—forces quite often beyond the knowledge or control of the parents—influence their children mightily.

It shows that family conflicts may seriously imperil the physical and psychological well-being of the very many troubled middle-aged parents for whom this book has been written.

And it introduces the frequently hurt and perplexed parent to effective and constructive ways of approaching and resolving these problems.

CHAPTER 1

UNDERSTANDING MIDDLE-AGED PARENTS AND THEIR ADULT PROBLEM CHILDREN

Nobody ever told me that being a parent was a lifetime job.

Introduction

The profound changes in American life over the last five decades have generated problems that earlier generations of parents did not have to face. As a consequence many middle-aged parents have seen their relationships with their adult children grow awkward, uncomfortable, marred by tension and anger. Since they have had little or no opportunity to learn the details of these newly minted puzzles, or to acquire experience in dealing with them, today's middle-aged parents often find such conflicts difficult, frustrating, and seemingly insoluble. Here are some examples:

Steve, a bright, ingratiating, and apparently stable 28-year-old, graduated with honors from the university five years ago. He looked for work for about six months, but gradually gave up the search. Now, four years later, he still lives at home, dependent on his parents. They feel let down, worried, cheated, and helpless at his lack of initiative, his inertia, his parasitic self-content.

John and Emily are in their early sixties. Their youngest child, Marge, had a turbulent adolescence marked by drug abuse and repeated runaways. When she reached her twenties she seemed to settle down, married, and almost immediately had a child. She and her husband split up after two years. The husband left her and not long afterwards Marge moved away, thrusting the child, then two, into the care of the grandparents. They felt that they had no alternative but to accept and look after the youngster, although its presence has caused them much physical, psychological, and economic strain and has shattered their retirement plans.

*

Jack, Barry's father, is a hard-working, high-achieving man who, through determined effort and much perseverance has achieved well-deserved recognition in university teaching. Barry, intellectually gifted, attended a good university where he made barely passing grades. When he finally graduated he drifted from one job to another until he found steady employment as a firefighter. Jack cannot understand or accept Barry's lackadaisical attitude toward work and his willingness to stick with a blue-collar occupation. He feels ashamed and somehow to blame for what he considers to be his son's lack of ambition.

To the sorts of problems outlined above—the uncut cord that binds Steve to his parents, John and Emily's dangling grandchild, Barry's "falling short" of Jack's expectations—others can be added. There are the well-meaning, but meddlesome grandparents, incomprehensible "lifestyles," gay children, children caught up in religious or political extremism, children addicted to drugs or alcohol, children with disabling illnesses, and children who get into financial, legal, or sexual scrapes. These are some of the problems now prevalent—predicaments often new enough that there is little accumulated experience or "folk wisdom" to guide their victims. Indeed, many parents feel humiliated to admit that they suffer such difficulties, not realizing that problem children may be found everywhere, plaguing very many similarly reticent and troubled mothers and fathers. Problems with adult kids are as American as apple pie.

Intergenerational Conflict and You

Despite the growing severity and frequency of problems involving adult children and their parents, surprisingly little has been written about them. However, much has been said and written about generational conflict and its causes and characteristics, which conflict is rooted in differing assumptions about the way in which one's life ought to be lived.

The potential for such disagreement exists in most families. The Gallup Poll, which regularly looks into social, political, economic, and religious attitudes of Americans, finds that on some issues individuals in the 18–29 year age bracket and those 50 years of age or older agree closely. On others (attitudes about premarital sex, abortion, equal rights, legalizing homosexuality, greater emphasis on self-expression, marijuana use, work, and authority), Gallup finds that there are gross differences between the generations. It is out of these differences that conflict can arise.

The actual disagreements are intensified by false conclusions the two generations reach about one another. Each group believes that the other holds more extreme views than it actually does. Adult children are much less liberal on social issues than their parents think; the parents are less conservative on those same issues than the children believe.

How You Can Avoid or Minimize Problems with Adult Children

In hindsight most middle-aged parents would agree that—of all the tasks they took on—the one for which they were least well-prepared was that of parenting. One expert sardonically says: "Most people are no more qualified to be parents than they are to be orthodontists."

The feeling of inadequacy that most parents harbor explains their readiness to accept the blame when something goes sour with their kids. The anguished question, "Where did I go wrong?" is the first one the counselor is likely to hear when consulting with a parent who has a problem offspring.

There is no way to dodge or anticipate all of the problems that may crop up during child-rearing. Parents simply cannot foretell the future, so that any prescriptions about how optimally to bring up children rests on their own experiences as children, along with their shaky personal forecasts about what the future world will be like and what kinds of qualities will serve the child best or most effectively when he or she enters that world.

Since difficulties are bound to occur, parents will be best served by accepting the prospect that they will crop up. Then, when problems do in fact materialize, the parents can focus on managing them in the least damaging way by observing three principles: Act directly—act dispassionately—act without delay.

Acting directly entails nothing more than approaching the child and airing the problematic matter openly, whatever it may be. Many—perhaps most—individuals do not enjoy confrontations and would much rather see matters improve without having to become directly involved. They would prefer to work behind the scenes—to manipulate the situation so that the desired change occurs without them having to suffer the tension and stress that may ensue. This evasive tactic should be avoided. It usually doesn't fool anybody; it may backfire by intensifying the problem, blowing it out of proportion; and, worst of all, it is dishonest.

Being dispassionate calls on the parents to manage or control their feelings—feelings that will almost certainly run high and deep. Putting a brake on them will help the parents to express their own concerns rationally while allowing the child every opportunity to state his or her side of the matter fully and freely. This commitment to reason keeps parents from blowing up or making up their minds in advance about what should or should not be done.

Moving on a problem without delay is self-evidently important. Prompt action will keep the problem from either growing larger or taking on an exaggerated importance. And it will also nip stress and tension—and their destructive consequences—in the bud.

How to Tell Whether You Really Have a Problem

It is often difficult to know exactly what the problems between middle-aged parents and their adult children are. The situation is invariably complex, and it is perceived in somewhat different terms by those involved, so that definition of the scope, nature, or severity of the problem is what is initially required. Parts 2–4 of this book treat the issue carefully, analyzing what constitutes a specific problem, when it occurs, and who in fact really suffers the problem.

Two types of adult child vs middle-aged parent problems emerge from this analysis. First, there are those troubles that are shared or held in common—that is, they are recognized as problems for both the parent and the child. Second, there are individual vexations that constitute a problem only for parent or child. A homosexual son whose sexual orientation concerns both him and his parents constitutes a shared problem; a homosexual son whose sexual orientation concerns only his parents amounts to an individual parental problem. The present book deals only with shared problems of parents and children or the individual problems of parents. It does not go into the ways in which children may effectively contend with their own individual difficulties.

Our general consideration of problems in the abstract then gives way to specific descriptions of real quandaries that parents and children (or parents alone) have experienced. The examples have been drawn from my more than 30 years' experience as a teacher and counselor helping troubled young adults and their parents. This experience has shown that both inter- and intrapersonal conflicts feed on the inability or unwillingness of the antagonists to deal openly and dispassionately with one another, and are often made worse by a failure to consider the rights and responsibilities of others—or oneself. This failure not only creates unnecessary troubles; it also intensifies them, making them more painful and persistent than they need to be. Accordingly, methods for opening the lines of communication and locating the source and site of the trouble are presented throughout the book.

How to Stop Taking the Blame
for Your Adult Child's Actions

Child-rearing has a uniquely powerful capacity to bring on feelings of doubt and to undermine one's self-confidence. Thus, if something goes sour with a child, these well-tended feelings provide fertile soil in which the seeds of blame and guilt may take root and flourish.

This parental stampede to take responsibility for all their children's failings rests on a faulty assumption. It attaches all of the responsibility to environmental influences—and to a single set of environmental influences at that. Though early experience within the family plays a considerable part in shaping the adult personality, other forces that are almost completely outside the control of the parents also play a significant role in the child's development.

Heredity—the genetic factor—represents one important and uncontrollable contributor to the makeup of the adult persona. Beyond such obvious physical qualities as race, sex, height, weight, handedness, and color of eyes and hair, heredity has something fundamental to say about predisposition to certain illnesses, level of intelligence, basal metabolic rate, overall level of activity, the presence of certain specialized abilities, and the like. Nothing that the individual becomes stands independent of the genetic inheritance. This significant bequest from our forebears is a matter of chance and can only be slightly modified by environmental manipulation.

Socialization is the other important, but usually not well-controlled, factor contributing strongly to a child's persona. Self-blame errs by playing down the existence and the potency of the many influences outside the family. School and church exist to mold the student or communicant along certain lines. Work has much to say about how individuals view and conduct themselves. Peers exert enormous influence on significant aspects of behavior, setting and enforcing standards for taste, dress, recreation, moral conduct, and the like.

Peer pressure is especially hard to resist and by definition stands outside the sphere of influence of the parents. The resourceful self-blamer has an answer for this, of course. "If I had done a good job of bringing up Janie, she never would have caved in to that sort of pressure," the parent is likely to say. For this die-hard, the work of the psychologists Stanley Milgram and Solomon Asch may be instructive.

Milgram showed that most individuals, when placed under severe authoritarian pressure to conform, administered what they believed were extremely painful and just possibly lethal electric shocks to other individuals in order to get them to carry out a task correctly. Even though they believed (quite wrongly) that the other person, the learner, felt acute pain, the great majority of "teachers" persisted in the experiment. Only a few refused to continue administering the high-voltage shocks and their verbatim accounts suggest that these drop-outs had some built-in ability to resist authority.

Asch showed that peer pressure is extremely powerful in forcing individuals to make judgments that directly and unmistakably contradict their own perceptions. In his experiment only a few individuals did not succumb to the pressure to make judgments obviously at odds with the facts. Of these unusual individuals, Asch said that they were able to oppose without compromising their sense of personal worth only because their noncompliance with peer pressure did not threaten their own feelings of integrity. It follows from this that closer supervision or guidance from parents, because it makes it more difficult to abide by one's own experiences, would have the unintended result of making children more rather than less susceptible to peer pressure.

Although the problems that some adult children bring back to their parents may indeed be laid at the parents' door, open-and-shut cases of parental culpability are uncommon. Assuming blame for a problem, whether or not the circumstances warrant such an admission, will not change the problem or make it go away. Following the line of reasoning that begins "If I had only done thus and so, then this never would have happened," is a seductive but useless activity. One can never know what might have occurred if something different had been tried at some earlier time in the upbringing of the child. Things might have turned out the same, worse, or better. Guilt and self-reproach force the groundless conclusion that different tactics would have had less painful results.

The parental tendency to take responsibility for problems of or with adult children has one additional flaw. Luxuriating in guilt will often prevent or delay the development of solutions to the difficulty.

The eagerness of parents to assume guilt for their children's plights is easy enough to understand. Parents generally see themselves as "responsible" for their children and are thus accustomed to making amends for their misbehaviors. Parents also care deeply about their children—not always, of course, but most do, most of the time—and willingly make sacrifices and accept heavy obligations for the sakes of their children. Parental self-blame is another and especially ineffective way of easing the child's path. Even though a parent might happily assume responsibility for a problem, that action will not miraculously free the child of it. No matter how hard the parents try—and no matter what tactics they use—an adult child is ultimately left to face the consequences of his or her actions. The problem stays put.

How Problems with Adult Children Can Hurt You

The problems that adult children bring home—or that their parents insist on taking responsibility for when they have neither the right nor the need to do so—can have devastating side effects on all involved. The feelings of disappointment, the sense of failure, the thwarted hopes and expectations, the upset of personal plans—all undermine the sense of competence and well-being of the parent. These feelings can lead to the onset of severe, crippling psychological or physical complaints. Knowing that these kinds of parent–child problems can impair health and greatly erode feelings of worth and potency is essential to formulating courses of action that will address them as forthrightly and effectively as possible.

What You Can Do to Meet Problems Coolly and Constructively

The final section of this book presents a general method and series of strategies to follow in identifying, analyzing, and dealing with problems middle-aged parents may encounter with their grown children. The procedure—a rational, order-ly decision-making process—rests on four assumptions:

First, most parent–child dilemmas carry a great deal of emotional freight, a burden that often interferes with the de-velopment of productive, creative, and mutually satisfactory solutions. Any procedure that promotes a rational and or-derly approach to a problem will prove effective and holds the greatest promise of constructive action.

Second, each possibly useful method of dealing with a given problem will have its own unique set of consequences. Attempted solutions that do not work out often fail because of unforeseen complications. It is crucially important to de-cide in advance what consequences are acceptable. Is getting rid of a problem worth risking the loss of the child's esteem or of earning its actual enmity? And, among those solutions that are acceptable, it is essential to select that set of consequences offering promise of either the greatest gain or the least harm.

Third, suggested procedures and methods of analysis are fine in their way, but effective problem-solving requires real work. The method not only has to be studied and understood —it has to be tried, put into action. To help in reaching this goal, Chapter 19 will provide a programmed exercise in which the reader is asked to analyze, chart the consequences of, and select from among the available alternatives a course of action that gives promise of being the most successful, con-structive, or fruitful one conceivable. Unhappily, but realisti-cally, since many of the conflicts that plague parents and their adult children are enormously complex and thorny, this pro-cedure may occasionally lead only to adoption of the prospec-tively least unsuccessful, least unconstructive, or least un-fruitful alternative.

Fourth, the problem may sometimes be beyond the capac-ity of the parent to manage unaided. It is important to be able to recognize when that is true and to have the fortitude, as well as the ability, to locate the right kind and amount of outside help when the necessity for it becomes evident. The final chapter is devoted to this topic. In it I argue that recognizing and acting on the perceived need for assistance is an indication of individual strength rather than weakness. Beleaguered parents need to know when, why, where, and to whom they can turn for help, what forms helping relationships may take, and what they can realistically expect in the way of results.

Chapter 2

HOW DID ALL THIS HAPPEN?

Times change; people change.

Introduction

By presenting brief sketches of a very few of the many cataclysmic changes that have occurred in this country in the last half century, I hope to provide here an idea of the range and power of the forces that have drastically redefined the relationship between grown children and their parents during the same period. This brief social history is not meant to be complete—everyone knows that change has been profound and that its rate is accelerating. The impact of these changes on parent–child relationships is not quite so evident, however, and the discussions that follow merely highlight a few of the shifts and give an idea of the wide range of effects they have exerted. For any example given here, the thoughtful reader will no doubt be able to supply a dozen more.

At the heart of the problems that today's middle-aged parents are experiencing with their adult children is one inescapable fact: the world that the parents knew and tried to pass along to their children no longer exists. Middle-aged parents, when they were children, lived in a social universe as different from that of their children as their own had been different from the world of Julius Caesar.

17

Let's take 1930 as a convenient birthdate for the representative of today's middle-aged generation. Back then, radio
was in its infancy; television was a Sunday Supplement fan-
tasy; talking pictures were still on the way; space travel was a
fiction writer's dream; it was impossible to buy a legal alcoholic drink anywhere in the United States; there were no park-
ing meters.

A substantial proportion of the homes had neither elec-
tricity nor running water; refrigerated air conditioning did
not exist; the flies on trousers buttoned; women, who had had
the right to vote for only a short decade, did not wear trousers.

Diphtheria, tuberculosis, whooping cough, scarlet fever,
measles, mumps, rubella, and polio were pandemic. There
was no birth control pill or morning after foam; abortion was
legal only under the most extraordinary and stringent of circumstances.

Nylon, most of the other synthetic fabrics, and plastics
had not found their way to the marketplace.

These changes, at which the preceding list only begins to
hint, have erected massive barriers to understanding between
the generations. Each is caught in its own web of circumstances, its own world—and each of these worlds holds much
that is strange and mysterious to the other. The result? Separation, and the opening of physical, social, and psychological
gulfs between the generations.

Individual Change
and Conflict Between Generations

Individuals, in whatever social circumstance they are
found, inevitably pass through characteristic stages of development. These stages have always been accompanied by periods of stress and conflict. And of course they do not stand

independent of their sociocultural setting—an adolescent American boy, unlike an African Maravi youth, would not be ceremoniously expelled from home and left to fend for himself on a certain day when the signs and portents are right.

Erik Erikson, the psychiatrist, conceives of eight "Ages of Man" and describes them as a series of interdependent stages that include many psychosexual, physical, and cognitive changes (and their attendant tensions and conflicts). Each "Age" presents its own special hurdle; the way in which it is surmounted will be reflected in the later development of the individual.

Parents and children are each, at the same time, growing, adapting, adjusting. The problems that different individuals in various of Erikson's Ages encounter at any given moment are different—the six- or seven-year-old may be struggling with feelings of competence, while the child's parents are trying to cope with the burden that entry into the fourth decade of life imposes. These different but concurrent crises of parents and their children, born of developmental change, are also accompanied by changes in the society itself that occur regardless of what is happening to the individual.

Knowing all about such developmental stages will not make them vanish—they must of course be lived through. Simply understanding that they are fixed elements in the life processes of all persons, and that individuals of different ages may be striving to resolve different dilemmas at the same time, may itself help to smooth over some misunderstandings between children and parents. The middle-aged mother, aware of her own moments of despair, and also aware that her adult daughter inhabits another psychological space in which she is working through the nature and meaning of her relationships, can use this knowledge to respond with understanding and compassion when in fact a problem with the daughter surfaces.

Social Change and the Conflict Between Generations

Individual patterns of development can grow very confused in the swift tides of change now running in society at large. A middle-aged parent whose early background comes as close to that of Rome in the first century as it does to the conditions of the moment can be forgiven feelings of bemusement when confronted with such phenomena as talking automobile seat belts or Michael Jackson. Change is occurring rapidly in all aspects of American life and wherever it happens, it affects relationships between the generations.

Technological Change

At the heart of all of the other social developments that have occurred in this country in the past half-century is the extraordinary growth in its technology—the direct effects of this growth are obvious and everywhere. Satellites. Television. Agribusiness. The H-bomb. Leather-skinned tomatoes. Styrofoam. Personal computers. Smog. Technology may be thanked for making American lives far more easy, comfortable, affluent, faster-paced, complex, hazardous, and stressful than they were back in the 30s.

In addition to affecting what people wear and eat, and to influencing how and where they work and live, technology has transformed how and what citizens think, believe, value, and enjoy. Other changing aspects of American life—political, demographic, economic, educational, and even recreational—were triggered by explosive technological change. Let's take developments in medical practice as one indicator of the impact of technology.

Fifty years ago medical treatment was largely directed toward alleviating symptoms; that is, the doctor, carrying a limited range of medicines around in a little black bag, could only relieve, or somewhat reduce, the aches, pains, and fever that accompanied illness. The disease itself and its course were invulnerable and the body was left to accomplish its own healing.

Since 1930, however, many once-common diseases have largely been brought to heel and eradicated. Typhoid, diphtheria, and acute poliomyelitis, for all practical purposes, no longer exist in the United States. Scarlet fever and measles respond quickly to medication, so that their once-dreaded consequences have vanished. Smallpox was declared eradicated in 1979. The incidences of tuberculosis and leprosy have dropped dramatically as those afflictions have been brought under medical control.

The little black bag has been replaced by the *Physician's Desk Reference*, a tome that, in its current 2016 page edition, lists many thousands of available drugs, their applications in a wide variety of complaints and illnesses, their manufacturers, and both their direct and side effects.

Medical advances have alleviated much of the anxiety parents commonly experienced as a part of the process of rearing children. What parent under the age of 30 knows the awful dread that went with the polio season before Salk and Sabin? And even when there is only anxiety, this too can be eased by resorting to an arsenal of psychotropic drugs.

The revolution in the efficacy of medical treatment has had its parallel in the growth of knowledge about and the ability to direct and control normal bodily activities. The most significant of these biomedical breakthroughs has been the discovery of means to control the process of human reproduction. The pill and other new methods of avoiding pregnancy have exerted a profound influence on attitudes toward and feelings about sexual activity, reducing much apprehension, anxiety, and guilt, especially in connection with premarital sex. The legalization of abortion has also contributed to the freeing of attitudes about sex, especially in the younger age groups. Today's 50-year-old grew to young adulthood dur-

ing a time when premarital sexual activity was strongly condemned and was subject to a variety of social sanctions. Pregnancy out of wedlock, which at that time could be legally ter-
minated only under the most extraordinary circumstances,
stigmatized all those involved—the principals, their families,
and, of course, the child.

This disapprobation has given way to the "new morality," which takes a much more tolerant view of sexual activity
and of bearing and rearing children outside of marriage.
"Meaningful relationships" are common and accepted matter-of-factly by the majority of young adults. Their parents
often do not display the same degree of permissiveness, since
their attitudes about premarital or extramarital sex and cohabitation are tempered by their early training and the conditions that prevailed when they were entering adulthood.
Medical advances have made the "new morality" possible
and with its appearance have sprung up a rash of intergenerational conflicts growing out of disagreements about the place,
purpose, meaning, and signifance of sexual activity.

Many other attitude-affecting medical advances could be
cited—the extension of life through technological means,
organ transplants, the mechanical maintenance of bodily
functions that permits physicians to intervene directly in
processes that, not too long ago, were completely out of reach.
These developments, along with the recent appearance of
"test tube" babies and recombinant genetic research, challenge traditional assumptions about the significance and
meaning of conception, birth, life, and even death.

This sketchy account of the impact of medical developments on contemporary life describes only one small aspect of
the overwhelming influence of technological change on contemporary life. Simply put, technological advances have radically transformed the physical conditions of daily life. They
have also mediated shifts in personal values and attitudes.
They have prompted a kind of mobility that has transformed

the family structure and made a pawn of the American worker; they have created a consumer-based society in which disposability and built-in obsolescence have supplanted the older values of "use it up, wear it out, make it do." And, finally, they have created a society in which the qualities of patience, moderation, and thriftiness are frequently irrelevant, if not actually subversive.

This is not to say that technological and scientific development have been destructive; life is—or can be—easier, fuller, freer, more interesting, and more complex and stimulating now than it was a few decades ago. For much of that we owe a debt to technology. But these changes have had their costs, too, working to distance adult children even more sharply from their middle-aged parents.

Social Factors

There have been equally significant changes in the entire social fabric of the United States in the past half century.

The transformations in the status of youth and in the institution of marriage in American life over that period barely hint at the enormous upheaval that has occurred.

The middle-aged segment of today's society was taught that "Children should be seen and not heard." As children they were expected to be dependent, polite, obedient, respectful, and quiet when in the presence of adults. They may have disliked or resented what they were called on to do or be, but that was the role they were stuck with and they played it out —grudgingly, resentfully perhaps, but they did it.

Assumptions about the role and nature of children and about the preferred methods of child-rearing have changed, with directive, authoritarian practices giving way to more permissive or child-centered ones. This shift led eventually to a redefinition of the place of children. No longer were they simply regarded as small adults and dealt with accordingly. One result has been the evolution of a special judicial system for youthful offenders considered to be qualitatively different from adults. Juvenile misconduct is now judged, punished, and corrected by a newly developed set of rules and procedures.

These switches in fundamental attitudes have made possible the emergence of a separate and distinct "youth culture." Though there has always been a youth culture of sorts, what has evolved in the United States and, to a lesser extent elsewhere, is a quantum leap beyond the youth culture of the past. What we now have is a subculture with its own standards of behavior and mores, with its own distinct attitudes, music, dress and appearance code, and with its own special vocabulary and rituals.

One enduring result of this trend has been the walling off of young people from adults, creating a sort of intrafamily ghetto of the young. In an attempt to breach this wall, the voting age was lowered to eighteen, but that move has had its own ironies. Young people, in the aggregate, are much less inclined to vote than their parents or grandparents, although it was at first thought that they would be enthusiastic participants in the electoral process. Moreover, while the voting age has been lowered, the legal age for drinking has been raised to 21 in many places, so that eighteen year-olds are told that they can help to elect a president, but that they must wait another three years to do something so really important as buying a drink legally.

Young adults hold attitudes and values that can and often do differ from those of their parents. Differences in outlook over rights and responsibilities—whether they refer to such trivial matters as the manner of dress or hairstyle, or to more substantive ones, such as the kinds of commitments that inhere in interpersonal relationships—are sources of distance, dissension, and conflict between the groups.

Marriage is a particularly apt example of institutional change: Age at marriage has gradually increased; marriage often follows a substantial period of cohabitation; marriage is much more likely to occur between individuals from different religious or ethnic backgrounds; and the marriage is much less prone to endure than was formerly the case. Older people are likely to be sardonically amused at a "white wedding" or a "honeymoon" involving a couple who have been living together, sometimes for years. To them such actions cheapen or mock the symbolic meaning of the custom.

Half a century ago divorce (or dissolution of marriage, to use its emotionally more neutral synonym) was relatively uncommon; now nearly four in ten marriages end in divorce and the number of divorces has quadrupled annually since 1960. The increasing incidence of dissolution of marriage has largely removed the stigma attached to the process itself among younger individuals. This is not so true for many middle-aged parents, who are likely to have a better track record for marital endurance, who have emotional ties that divorce disrupts, and who may be (or fear that they may be) forced to take on the responsibility of rearing their grandchildren—or, alternatively, who fear that they will lose touch with them.

Among young adults, relationships, whether sanctified by marriage or not, are fragile and, by their parents' standards, short-lived. The typical marriage endures for seven years. The parental generation was taught to regard marriage as a once-in-a-lifetime commitment. Though this belief did not entirely mesh with experience—marriages did wind up in the courts, even then—a divorce hinted at impropriety. Young adults may hope for stability and permanence in their marital relationships, but they are more aware of the risks and realities of the institution and, by virtue of this knowledge, are often better prepared to deal with the wreckage when a breakup occurs. What marriage is, what it entails, and what it means summon quite disparate views from middle-aged parents and their grown issue. In these differences lies a multitude of possibilities for misunderstanding and conflict.

Demographic Factors

Technological and social change have brought about many sweeping changes in the demographic characteristics of today's population, and these changes, occurring within the lifetime of our current crop of middle-aged parents, have had a most divisive effect. With the enormous impact of technology on agriculture, for instance, the rural–urban distribution of the population has shifted markedly. There are only one-half as many farms today as there were in 1940; more than 25% of the individuals still on farms are over 55 years of age, and the absolute number of individuals living on farms has fallen by nearly two million workers—this despite a phenomenal increase in the absolute, as well as the relative, value of farm products.

Partly as a result of this change there has been a great cityward migration. Whites moved, first to the cities and then, when they could, to the suburbs; blacks left the rural south to find work in the industrial cities of the northeast and middle west. More recently, most of the larger cities have been losing population and the composition of their residents has been shifting so that the minority poor constitute an increasingly greater proportion of city dwellers.

The distribution of the population as a whole has also been undergoing changes, particularly by its wholesale gravitation toward the Sun Belt. This has happened partly because industries have relocated there, and partly as a result of personal retirement strategies. From 1940 to 1980 the population of the western states grew at a rate of 307%; the figure for the country as a whole was 172%.

The characteristics of the work force are also shifting radically. Not only are there many fewer workers in agriculture, but blue-collar workers are also becoming relatively scarcer, while the number and percentage of people engaged in white collar and service occupations continues to rise. From 1960 to

1980 the proportion of the population engaged in service occupations increased more than one-third and those in white collar jobs went up by something over ten percent.

The American family is not what it used to be, either. Though it is customary to think of it as consisting of a married couple with two children, this view does not fit the data. Nuclear families in which the husband is the sole wage earner now constitute fewer than one in five. Almost half of American households now contain only two members. The single-parent family constitutes about one-fifth of the households and the proportion of people who live in families at all has been on the decline since 1940. The average household in 1940 had 3.7 members; in 1980, 2.7. These changes reflect a number of trends in the society, one of which is a shift in the attitude toward having children. Many young couples elect not to have children, in some cases because children entail responsibilities they are not willing to accept, in others because they believe that adding to the population is morally wrong.

The single-parent family reflects the increasing divorce rate or, less often, the decision of an unmarried parent to keep the child born out of wedlock. This last development slightly counters the widespread use of medical abortion which, in 1982, came to 1.6 million. During that year there were 426 abortions per 1000 live births and 28.8 per 1000 women. Legal termination of pregnancy by abortion for all practical purposes did not exist in 1940.

The decision to limit family size largely results from women's increased presence in the workplace. In 40 years, the number of women in the labor force has tripled. In 1940, only 24% of the work force was women; in 1980, it was 43%. With both partners employed, the level of affluence of the family unit has risen and this readily noticed improvement in the material situation of double income families tends to be habit-forming.

These and a host of other factors—the growth in size of
the young adult and middle-aged groups in our society, the
increasing ghettoization according to age, and so on—have
eroded previous expectations of order, stability, coherence,
and permanence. The nuclear family can no longer hold or
transmit these values effectively, and this inability is especially evident to the younger generations. Older folks may
not see it quite so clearly and this difference in perception is
itself another source of intergenerational misunderstanding,
as are different ideas about the character and meaning of
work, shifts in the composition and location of the work force,
and the growth of affluence.

Economic Factors

Economic factors have also weighed in to add to the split
between young and old. The growth in the relative size of
large-scale enterprises has consolidated production and made
the activities of a small number of extremely large enterprises
significantly more important.

This growth in scale reaches into all areas—agribusiness
has all but taken over the family farm; shopping malls with
their merchandising chain tenants have supplanted small,
locally owned variety, grocery, and department stores; newspaper chains widen their holdings while local publications
die; huge conglomerates are spawned. This ballooning,
which is more than matched by the growth in size and complexity of all levels of government, has replaced what the
older generation perceived as an intensive and more human
system of production and distribution with an ever more
extensive, depersonalized, bureaucratized one.

The ethic of scarcity and the belief in the need to husband
resources has given way to a social construct based on a faith
in abundance and the need to consume and to exploit resources. Products are made to wear out or, worse, to become

obsolescent, to fall out of fashion and lose their desirability on that account. Consumer goods, from cars to clothing to chocolate, conform to the dictates of fashion.

The emphasis on consumption makes for waste, pollution, and squandering of resources. It encourages people to take no heed of the future, to live in and for the moment. This emphasis on immediacy of experience and gratification is one of the cardinal distinctions between the lives and values of older and younger folk.

Another economic "factor" is the gross difference in the level of affluence that the two generations have experienced. The middle-aged generation had to weather the most troubled period in the economic history of the United States—the Great Depression of the 1930s. These hard times had an indelible effect on the outlook of that generation, making work and economic security a matter of paramount importance.

After the 1930s the country passed into a period of armed conflict followed by an extended era of "good times" that has been interrupted only briefly by small recessions. Work has been plentiful; opportunities to move upward, economically or in status, were never better, and this boom period has continued until the late 1970s. Children who grew up in the 50s and 60s, lacking any experience of deprivation, had little reason to develop the economic fears and misgivings that haunted their parents. The optimism of these children contrasts starkly with the apprehensive, security-obsessed pessimism so characteristic of their parents.

Political Factors

Differences between adult children and their parents are also mirrored in the political picture. Despite the lowering of the legal voting age and access to the voting booth over the past fifteen years or so, the young, the economically disadvantaged, and ethnic minorities participate in the electoral process much less conscientiously than the older, more affluent, white segments of our society.

Young adults have been greatly influenced by the war in Viet Nam and the Watergate scandal. These complex and tragic affairs have eroded confidence in the electoral process and belief in the power of the individual to influence domestic or foreign policy. Cynicism and feelings of impotence underlie the failure of the young to have their say in the political life of the country.

Disillusionment with the electoral process also owes something to the fact that running for and gaining any political office has become so expensive that elections are in the hands of professional consultants and the pockets of big spenders. The experts use opinion polls and the media to sell the candidates. Voters, especially young voters who see political office seekers marketed like soap or dog food, retreat into resentment and apathy, convinced that he who giveth (to a political candidate) shall receive.

These feelings are abetted by a blurring of the distinction between candidates and parties that seems to have turned campaigning and governing into a process of scurrying from one hot issue to the next, of management by crisis. Persistent, long-term problems are shunted aside and little happens to encourage belief in the orderliness, coherence, or effectiveness of the system. "Big government" is seen by the American public as the single most serious problem confronting the country.

Faith in the political process and institutions, and in the power of voters to affect policies and events, has been deeply shaken. Even so, the over-50 generation continues to participate in the political rituals; younger voters, demoralized and disillusioned, in large part ignore them. As one writer puts it, "Cultural breakdown has reached the point of no return when the process of socialization no longer provides the new generation with coherent reasons to be enthusiastic about becoming adult members of the society."

Religious Factors

Loss of faith in political institutions and forms has been accompanied by a parallel decline in religious expression and conviction.

Though membership in a few of the more conservative Protestant sects has grown, participation in organized religion has fallen off sharply in the last half century. Despite the constitutional separation of church and state, the dominant values of the republic had long been rooted in the Protestant Ethic—a set of beliefs espousing the worthiness of thrift, self-denial, and hard work. As the validity of these assumptions came to be challenged by recurrent cycles of boom and bust, the importance of organized religion, the prime carrier of these prescriptions, declined and participation in religious activities fell off.

Here, too, the young have been more ready to abandon religion and this has set the generations apart. The parents, professing a set of beliefs to which their children cannot subscribe, find themselves hard-pressed to comprehend or accept life values their kids have and with which they, the parents, disagree profoundly.

The overall decline in religious involvement has been slightly countered by the rise in popularity of fundamental Christian belief and the emergence of ecstatic religious movements. Although this phenomenon has involved relatively few individuals, it has provoked a great deal of publicity and engendered more than its share of parent–child unhappiness and alienation.

Educational Factors

Education, too, has done its part to separate the generations. In 1940 the typical adult over the age of 25 had barely completed the equivalent of elementary school; in 1983 the average number of years of schooling had shot up to 12.6. In 1940, 49% of the 18-year-olds graduated from high school; by 1983 the figure had risen to 72%. In 1940, approximately 12% of high school graduates went on to college; now over 50% do.

Underlying this explosive growth is the faith that education pays off monetarily. In 1960 it was estimated that the average lifetime earnings of college graduates would be three times greater than those of individuals with only an elementary school education. Though this forecast would not be quite so true today, cultural "lag" is such that most people—parents and children alike—still consider higher education as the "Open, Sesame!" to better, higher-paying, secure careers.

Above and beyond the promise of a dollar payoff, education has taken on other functions. It has increasingly assumed responsibility for training and certifying individuals for slots in the industrial or governmental bureaucracies or the professions. It has also provided a "cooling out" function by offering an interlude between graduation from high school and entry into the labor force. The nagging and growing problem of unemployment or underemployment of the young has thus been somewhat alleviated by this emphasis on college training. In this role, education—or, more exactly, the fact of being in college—has exposed young people to and sometimes encouraged flirtation with new, unfamiliar ideas. Support for rights causes—minorities, women—originated and is particularly strong on campuses; the youth culture, the counterculture, and the radical movements of the 60s began there, as did the opposition to the Viet Nam war. Groups espousing all shades of opinion—from radical right to radical left—are found on most campuses; so are recruiters for youth religious movements. The colleges are home to a smorgasbord of ideologies, some of which have seriously alarmed, mystified, and threatened parents.

More years of schooling have become necessary as the technological revolution has advanced. Basic educational skills are needed to function in a labor market that calls for ever higher and more sophisticated levels of training. Or, so it is said. Actually, the amount of formal training required is often irrelevant to the demands of the job, but the educational requirement is kept because it will screen out some individuals, thus reducing the size of the pool of applicants. Imposing an educational requirement saves time and money for the prospective employer and probably does not injure the validity of the selection process greatly.

The dramatic increase in the difference in number of years of schooling completed by the generations has driven a wedge between them. Education, generally, is associated with the development of more liberal, less authoritarian values, so that the strong push to have more education may have the unintended result of putting children and parents on opposite sides of the ideological fence.

The main problem with education as it affects the relationship between parents and children has been education's recent difficulty in delivering on its implied promises. At one time a college degree virtually assured entry into secure, socially valued, responsible, and remunerative work. The huge increase in the supply of college-trained individuals has made finding work appropriate to the level of training much more difficult. This has frustrated and disappointed both parents and children whose expectations for the future have been thwarted or downgraded. Thus a growing class of overeducated (or underemployed) persons has lately come onto the scene. Parents find it difficult to understand or accept that their children are employed at levels and in jobs below their education, falling short of the ideals and expectations held out for them. Faced with the fact that the efforts and sacrifices they have made on behalf of their children have not paid off, some parents become bitter, resentful, or openly critical of school and child. Confronted with a shrinking or non-existent market for their skills and training, some young adults feel cheated and misled; others give up trying to enter the labor market at any level, electing to remain at home. The children who stay in the nest, living off the parents long past the time when they were supposed to be out fending for themselves, represent a growing and especially vexing problem for many families.

CHAPTER 3

HOW CONFLICT WITH THEIR ADULT CHILDREN CAN HARM MIDDLE-AGED PARENTS

Introduction

As we have seen, today's adult children and their middle-aged parents have divergent experiences, expectations, tastes, and attitudes. That these basic differences often result in the kinds of misunderstandings that have triggered so many new and largely unprecedented intergenerational problems is hardly surprising.

Though there is no good time for trouble, the kinds of problems that adult children bring home to their parents—or the problems that parents insist on assuming when they have no business in doing so—strike members of the older generation at an especially vulnerable period in their lives.

Erik Erikson reminds us that the older generation is, after all, dependent on the younger one. Adulthood, the next to the last of his eight developmental stages, is taken up mainly with preparing and guiding the succeeding generation. Maturity, the very last Age, is ideally represented by persons who have the satisfaction of knowing that things—and people—have been looked after effectively, that everything has turned out satisfactorily.

When the next succeeding generation—the grown children of middle-aged parents—gives signs of being insecurely established or poorly guided, or when neither things nor people appear to have been taken care of adequately, the older generation is forced to grapple with what can easily be taken as its failure. This helps to account for many of the agonies of self-reproach that we see everywhere accompanying problems between these generations.

Middle age is seen as a settling-in period, a time when the responsibilities associated with child-rearing have, for better or for worse, been discharged. By then the children ought to be out of sight and largely out of mind. There will be freedom to do things long-postponed and, with the children no longer dependent, perhaps the means to do them. One expects to settle down, grow comfortable, have more time and opportunity to indulge oneself, and at last to relax and enjoy what has been so long denied or deferred.

The middle-aged person has probably gone about as far as he or she can go occupationally, functions competently and comfortably at work, and has adjusted tolerably to job, family, and the other aspects of life.

Middle age is not an idyll, of course. The looks may have fled, and with the looks some of the energy and stamina. Middle age brings with it the insistent reminder of one's own mortality—bad tidings in a society that worships youth. Psychological change may occur; a more sober or somber outlook, more firmly fixed ideas, less adaptability, less patience. Having to confront unwanted and unanticipated difficulties at the same time that one is growing more aware of and preoccupied with one's own life processes is enough to distress anyone. The stress and tension that accompany problems with adult children can precipitate major and totally unexpected troubles for middle-aged parents. Stressful conflicts with grown children can be hazardous to the patient's physical as well as emotional health.

The Stress of Life

Stress reactions are a routine aspect of life: they are essential to survival. Both agreeable and unpleasant events prove stressful. Marriage increases tension; so does divorce. Stress and its physiological companions help the organism—human or not—to adapt quickly to its surroundings. Yet, when the response to stress becomes extreme or prolonged, it may turn out to be maladaptive, actually causing illness. Problems and crises can have disagreeable consequences for the individual; the longer they remain unresolved, the more severe and lasting those consequences can be.

Stress can act indirectly to damage a person—if sufficiently extreme it can be lethal. And even if it does not have such drastic consequences, stress clearly correlates with a number of damaging physical symptoms.

A large number of investigations has established that stress, change, tension, transition—whatever the experience happens to be called—has long-lasting physical and psychological effects on the individual.

First, persons known to have experienced major amounts of stress and change are much more prone to illness than individuals comparable to them in all other respects who have not undergone such experiences.

Second, the more radical the change, the more grave may be the consequences. Not only does someone who has experienced considerable recent change have a greater likelihood of taking sick, but the greater or more taxing the change, the more severe any consequent physical ailment is likely to be.

Third, the stress that grows out of crises in family relationships is consistently among the most severe in terms of its impact on the individual. The death of a spouse has been found to be the most stressful life-change experience and it is the one most likely to have aftereffects; the death rate of widowers, for example, is forty percent higher in the year following bereavement than it is for comparable nonbereaved men. Other less serious family difficulties and crises rank high on the perceived level of severity and can precipitate a wide assortment of physical complaints.

Though there is a statistical relationship between stress and illness, that relationship is not immutable. After all, just because something stressful happens does not mean that unwelcome consequences will necessarily follow. The possibility is there of course, but it helps to remember that illness will not certainly result from stress in any individual case.

Stress and Physical and Psychological Illness

How does tension cause illness? Stress and life change affect the body chemistry. Indeed, any adaptation at all to events or circumstances upsets the hormonal balance. When disruptive conditions or events persist in one's life, calling for a high and continuing level of adaptation, these unrelenting demands on the body may either permit or actually produce physical ailments. It is as if the change, whatever it is, sets the machine to running at top speed, wearing out the component parts more rapidly, making progress more hazardous and causing breakdowns.

In addition to injury or a chilling variety of illnesses, stress may produce many other unpleasant consequences. Prolonged stress may accelerate the process of aging, affecting the appearance, the capacities, and the individual functions. It can exert profoundly disturbing sexual effects, upsetting the menstrual cycle in women, impairing potency and fertility in men, and destroying energy and desire in either gender.

Stress can also entail severe psychological–emotional consequences, as the following case illustrates:

Roger, sober, decent, hard-working, overprotective of his family, is a chronic worrier. He and his wife, Alicia, have two daughters. The older, Gracia, 22, bright, warm, and loving, but somewhat naive and sheltered, reveals in an intensely emotional scene that she is pregnant out of wedlock. Deeply distressed, upset, and shocked at the information, Roger stumbles out of the house, gets into his car, and drives off. Two days later he finds himself walking down the seamy skid row section of a city over 100 miles away from home. He has no recollection at all of how he got there, he cannot remember what he has done with the car, where he has stayed, or anything else that he has done in the 48 hours he has been gone. The car turns up in another town at some distance both from home and the city Roger in which "came to." It has a new dent in the left front fender, but no other signs of damage. It is parked, locked, on a side street. Roger still has the keys.

This incident in which the upset father went into a "fugue" or unconscious flight from reality illustrates an extreme reaction to stress. Though the matter was partially resolved by Gracia's decision not to have the baby, father, mother, and daughter all underwent a period of psychotherapy until the impact of these events was softened and eventually adjusted to.

Fortunately, most psychological reactions to radical life change, when they occur, are not so severe or frightening as the one Roger experienced. Roger's resulted from being brought face-to-face with a problem beyond his ability to manage. The solution, for him, was to get away from it by blanking out. This type of behavior (almost always less severe than the form it took with Roger) most often occurs when individuals are dealt more than they can handle. Apathy, withdrawal, or other behavior inappropriate to the situation can also result.

Another possible psychological reaction to a stressful situation includes focusing on one aspect or element of the problem, clutching to a small part of it rather than facing the whole.

> Cal and Lisa decide, after five years of marriage, that they have had enough and agree to a divorce. They have a four-year-old daughter and decide that Cal is to have custody of the child. Lisa's mother, greatly upset at the divorce, is unaware of the growing tendency for the male partner to take the children on separation or dissolution of marriage. She becomes obsessed with the decision and is unable to comprehend, much less accept, Lisa's explanations about the appropriateness of the action and the reassurances that the child will be with Lisa part of the time and that she, the grandmother, will not lose the opportunity to see, be with, and occasionally look after her granddaughter. She completely loses sight of the fact that three other individuals are going through a difficult period and could be greatly helped by a more supportive, constructive approach on her part. Instead, she continually returns to the custody issue, harping on it to Lisa as well as anyone else who will listen.

Ways of handling overload and the feelings of helplessness, conflict, and powerlessness that accompany it vary according to the individual. Some middle-aged parents trying to cope with their adult children exhibit the tendency to run backward in time, resurrecting a period in their and the child's lives when the parent had undisputed authority and control. This is seen when the parent suddenly starts treating the twenty-five-year-old child as if he or she were a disobedient six-year-old.

At other times parents oversimplify the problem, locking themselves into unrealistic solutions that ignore or deny the knottiness of the underlying situation. One mother kept saying of her gay son, "If he'd just marry and settle down with a nice girl, he'd be all right."

These reactions to change—flight, fixation, retreat, oversimplification—are ineffectual and sometimes counterproductive, but they are the best that the individual can come up with under the circumstances. However, other psychological disturbances often tag along.

Anxiety, one such consequence, has diffuse effects on its victims. Both conflict and confusion—not knowing what to do or what road to take when confronted with a problem—often prompt impulsive, ill-considered responses. Not seeing or not having any options, a frustrating state of affairs, can give rise to angry, aggressive, and even violent reactions directed at oneself or others.

These indirect emotional outcomes accompany efforts to deal with a problem that cannot be solved comfortably and readily out of past experience. When such a puzzler turns up the individual suffers a double dose of woe—psychological distress often accompanied by the physical side effects of stress, which can include headaches, stomach upsets, and similarly unwelcome bodily complaints.

Not the least danger occurs when a problem child's adult parents, driven by a situation that they cannot understand or manage, succumb to the inexorable pressure to do something. Some of our worst decisions—those that really come back to haunt us—are made when there is intense pressure to act with no obvious, logical way to head. The impulsive, irrational actions that so often result provide still further examples of the harmful psychological impacts produced by intergenerational problems.

How You Can Manage Stress, Conflict, and Their Consequences

In coping with stress, there are two routes you can take. First, you can do something about its cause directly, washing the aggravation or annoyance out of your system as the problem is solved or resolved. Second, if the problem defies solution, or if it cannot be attacked immediately and resolved swiftly, then you can learn to manage it, to live with it, and thereby to hold the effects of its stress to a minimum.

How does one go about the seemingly obvious task of dealing directly with a problem? At the outset, make sure that the situation is indeed a problem. All too often parents create or invent conflicts, or take problems personally, when they have no right to. When a difficulty does crop up, before acting you should first sit down someplace, quietly, by yourself and try to bring yourself to think calmly, clearly, and objectively about the problem. When you have reached that rational stage, you can then begin to figure out exactly what the trouble is (as nearly as you can understand it) and what part, if any, you play in the problem. If you cannot now state the problem or if, once stated, it does not make any sense to you, you should reanalyze it from the beginning. It is possible that the difficulty you thought confronted you really does not exist; or that you are somehow not making sense of the problem in your analysis. In either event, getting involved more deeply at that point would only complicate matters.

At this opening stage, you must decide whether you have any legitimate interest in the problem. Have you been asked to help? Is it honestly any of your affair? Have you anything to contribute? If you find yourself saying "No" to any of these questions, you can and should withdraw. All you will accomplish by jumping in where you are not needed or welcome is to make matters that much worse.

If you do conclude that a situation is not your problem (even though it may bother you a lot), how do you let it go? After all, it is your child who is in trouble. Turning your back and simply walking away is surely one of the harder tasks a parent may ever be called on to perform—but it is sometimes quite an essential one.

Despite the pain it may entail, you can cut yourself loose if you examine the likely consequences of your action, and particularly what it may mean to the child. You already know what it means to you—it amounts to desertion. But other matters may be considerably more important than your feeling that you have somehow failed to toss your child a lifejacket, especially when the truth of the matter may be that the child is not floundering and sees absolutely no need for your concern and your misguided efforts. Intervening in such circumstances may serve only to heighten and prolong the dependency of the child, while rendering the problem still more complex, long-lasting, and resistant to solution.

An important idea emerges here, one that parents have enormous difficulty in accepting. It is that saying "No," ruling yourself out, may be healthy for you as well as the child. If you can bring yourself to the point at which you can honestly say: "This problem does not involve me. I have no part in it." *or*, even more difficult, say "This is really your problem and it is up to you to handle it yourself," not only is the child liberated, but you too are freed. In particular, this action will liberate you from both the physical and psychological consequences of the problem. If you can honestly and comfortably declare that the problem does not concern you, and accept the corollary obligation not to intervene, your decision can be the most loving of acts—difficult and wrenching, no doubt, but ultimately loving because it releases you and the child from a bondage no longer appropriate to adults.

An employee of Alcoholics Anonymous, a woman now nearing sixty, once told me how her family had said "No."

I joined AA twenty-five years ago when my son was only five years old. We always had this big family Christmas get-together and I loved it so much. This one year they called it off. At least, that's what they told me, but I found out later that the celebration had been held. But I and my husband and son weren't invited because I always showed up half-drunk and by the time the thing was over I was completely blotto, an embarrassment to everybody. When I learned that my own family had cut me off because of what I was doing to myself and to them, I was crushed. Absolutely crushed. It opened my eyes, though. The next day I went to AA and I've been with them ever since. We have the Christmas celebration at our house now, but the best one ever was the one we went to the year after the year they didn't invite us.

The family saying "enough" in this case motivated the woman to do something about her problem even though the method used was abrupt and less straightforward than it might have been.

Now let us examine the situation in which you decide that a problem with your adult child cannot be put aside, that it does involve you in some way. Then the appropriate response is to act in such a manner that the effects of the problem are minimized for you. The problem should not be ignored since it will then only grow the more rapidly, fed by the imagination. Any such problem calls for action, but action of a particular kind. This is not the time to heed the old cry, "Don't just stand there. Do something!" by doing "something," or, as it so often turns out, almost anything, regardless of the chosen action's bearing on the problem and its potentially damaging effects.

Some sort of action is important, though, to keep the problem from worsening and to provide you, the parent, with a sense of movement and control. Getting to that stage entails talking with the other people involved and figuring out precisely what options exist. Intermediate steps sometimes need to be taken. If the difficulty should involve money or expense—a not uncommon complication when adult children are involved—then it may be necessary to figure out how the funds are to be secured if you choose to provide this kind of help. Then you will need to decide about recording the transaction, settling on repayment, and so on. Once the intermediate hurdles are cleared, the way is open to find out what specific alternatives you have. Sometimes none of them will be especially palatable and having to choose among distasteful options can cause vacillation. If your assessment has been thorough and careful, be aware that stalling because you have something disagreeable to do may be more stress-producing than actually carrying out the unrelished task. Hesitation, dithering, failing to resolve the conflict associated with a choice between unattractive alternatives will simply add to the likelihood of physical and psychological distress. If the problem is real, it will not go away, no matter how you agonize over it.

If you are backed into a corner where no avenues seem open to you, or where the actions under consideration are so bitter that you cannot take them, then you need to look for help and support elsewhere. Remember that nursing such a problem too long, wearing it like a hair shirt, will only spell trouble for you in the long run. Though there may be some perverse satisfaction in enduring such penitential suffering, there are other, more constructive ways of dealing with problems. Thus, it may be time to get help from someone else—be it other members of the family, or one of the many private or public counseling sources. Seeking such assistance can start you on the road to dealing concretely with the problem, and can also reduce the burden of dealing with it, permitting you to share the pain and difficulty with someone knowledgeable and sympathetic or, at the least, open and willing to hear and react to your side of the story. That, in itself, can keep disturbing matters from producing intolerable and potentially ruinous consequences for you and your child.

What has been said, until now, about managing stress, conflict, and reactions to them adds up to a process with a sequence of steps. Charted out it looks rather like the process shown in Figure 1.

Following the process outlined in the figure on the next page should show you, the troubled parent, what avenues remain open to you and which of these are least likely to harm you. Right now, the important points to remember are:

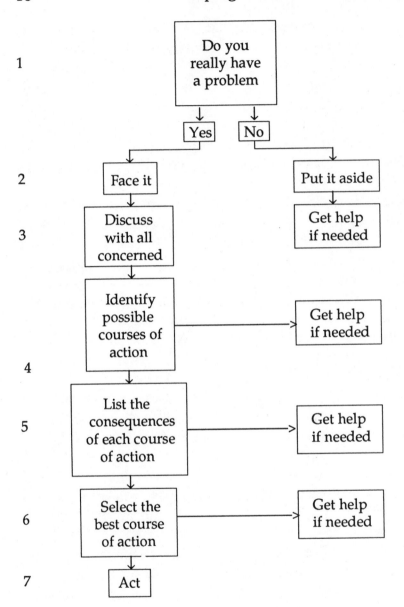

Fig. 1. The coping process—seven steps from problem to action

1. Problems that adult children bring home, or that you attempt to commandeer from them (whether or not you have any right or obligation to do so) can be deleterious to your physical and emotional health.

2. You are obliged to deal with a problem only when: (a) you choose to, or (b) it directly affects you.

3. Not becoming involved in a child's problem (keeping your distance or under certain circumstances refusing to become party to it) is often very difficult. Such benign noninvolvement is also, potentially, one of the most loving acts a parent can carry out.

4. Whatever you do should be done only after careful consideration. Impulsive, irrational actions undertaken largely because of an apparent need to do "something," understandable though they may be, frequently produce worse consequences than doing nothing at all.

5. If you are directly involved or cannot avoid being drawn into a problem, act promptly. This will often keep the problem under control and better your chances of dealing with it constructively. Prompt action will also minimize the kinds of physical and mental stress that so frequently accompany radical change.

6. Even if the options open to you are entirely unpalatable, selecting and acting on the least undesirable one may be better than delaying and fretting. Such indecisiveness, as we have noted, can be quite unhealthy and destructive.

7. If you cannot work out any suitable method for dealing with the problem on your own, seek help. This involves deciding whom the help is for, what kind is required, how much time and money can be devoted to it, how quickly it is needed, and so on. It *does not* involve judgments about what relatives, friends, or neighbors will think about your getting aid.

These steps in the process of dealing directly with inter-generational problems will help assure that destructive side effects—the erosion both of the physical and mental health, and of the well-being of the parents—are held to a minimum. All problems, whatever their nature, and whenever or wherever they are encountered, will have consequences of some kind—that much is inescapable.

Nowhere is it written that problems with grown children must be ignored until they are intolerable, overwhelming, unwieldy, and damaging. Following the steps outlined above will almost surely help you to keep them manageable, and minimally harmful to body and mind. It is a truism that the calendar is the great healer, and indeed many people seem to prefer drifting along in the hope that matters will take care of themselves. Though problems sometimes do resolve on their own, such a passive approach seems to me actually to encourage the growth of anxiety and its accompanying ill effects.

How You Can Handle Problems That Will Not Go Away

You can do a great deal at home to manage the stress and tension that inevitably accompany difficulties with adult children—or any other life problem for that matter. The process charted in the preceding section outlines one way of dealing constructively with significant life changes.

When it is not possible to attack the problem directly, or when measures taken to deal with a difficult situation fail, it may become necessary to do something about the symptoms of stress themselves.

Even though a problem with a child may stubbornly and upsettingly resist resolution, there are many ways in which you can learn to manage and control your own feelings and to be more comfortable with the situation, even when beset by the most trying circumstances.

Any of the strategies I have proposed, if followed, will offer some measure of relief. All remedies do have these things in common, however—they demand effort and fortitude. Solutions are there for the persistent inquirer, but they will not turn up unbidden. Moreover, troubled parents must be prepared to admit that their own feelings about a problem may be quite negative, and that they need to take definite steps if they are to control their upsetting and potentially harmful reactions.

One useful way the parent can cut such stress is to keep a busy schedule so that there is less opportunity to dwell on the problem. Participation in any one of many significant and demanding activities could diminish the significance of the crisis and thus reduce its potential for harm. Here are a few of the major possibilities:

Work, either paid or volunteer (for the retired), makes ongoing demands and provides rewards that help to sustain and nourish your sense of competence and worth in difficult times. And of course, one's opportunities for voluntary work are unlimited.

Hobbies provide an important avenue for relief from tension and stress, and should not be overlooked. What is suitable depends on individual preferences and the resources available. Handicrafts, gardening, and collecting are uncommonly helpful, among a long list of possibilities. There are organizations associated with most hobby activities that draw together those who share these common interests. Such groups can be especially important for the stimulation and camaraderie they offer.

Recreation, regardless of the form it takes, from extensive travel to softball or bingo one night a week, will help to break the routine and reduce preoccupation with one's troubles. There are enjoyable and diverting recreational pursuits available for everyone who may be involved in an otherwise all-consuming parent–child problem.

Regular exercise, appropriate to the age, interests, and capacities of the individual is an effective way of combating stress. Walking, jogging, or cycling can be done by almost everyone. Games or sports are useful diversions as well as sources of satisfaction in their own right. The motivated person can reap the benefits of exercise alone; those who need company in this endeavor can find it in adult education classes or such community-based organizations as the YMCA.

In addition to seeking out activities that distract or divert one's attention from even the quite serious problems, there are other ways of counteracting tension. Stressed individuals are prone to carelessness about what, when, or how often they eat. It has been shown that improper diet may contribute greatly to the severity of stress reactions. Following a sensible, nutritious diet has been found to be effective in reducing stress symptomatology. One of the first things parents who are in conflict with their adult children should do is look at what they themselves are eating and drinking, and be certain that they are sticking to a healthful diet. Alcohol or drug abuse (illegal or prescription) is particularly likely to happen during periods of acute stress. Excessive use of alcohol intensifies many of the feelings that grow out of tension; seeking solace in too much of the wrong kinds of food or drink carries dangers that are familiar to us all.

But perhaps the best way of reducing the stress that accompanies many problems with an adult child is for the concerned parent to talk to someone else about the situation. Simply being able to air the trouble openly to a sympathetic listener offers an important route to relief. The main obstacle here is the reluctance of many people to reveal or talk about problems they feel ashamed either of having or being unable to manage on their own. Those who are able to overcome this reticence due to inappropriate shame usually experience an enormous sense of relief.

Among those who have had training and experience in listening to and providing help with family conflicts are clergymen, physicians, and trained counselors (psychologists, family therapists, social workers, and other mental health professionals). Many people follow the practice of taking the problem initially to a clergyman or physician in order to develop suggestions about what to do next.

Revealing such intimate, personal problems to even a helpful stranger is extremely difficult, and it may thus be more comfortable, initially, to talk the matter over with a trusted friend or relative. This often helps to clarify one's thinking and define the problem more exactly. The strong sense of relief that accompanies such a sharing of the problem will still occur, and the disclosure may thus pave the way for seeking out long-term help.

Finally, many techniques have been developed that are specifically aimed at stress reduction. These may include simply learning how to relax periodically and/or rapidly when under stress. There are, in addition, exercises and meditative techniques that have been found effective in achieving and maintaining a more tranquil state. Other, more exotic methods of reducing stress and tension—hypnosis, biofeedback, or acupuncture—can be obtained from individuals trained in and competent to administer such treatments. In general, however, the strategies that one develops on one's own for dealing with stress are probably more effective than those supplied by outsiders. Activity, discussion, and relaxation are far better means of controlling stress symptomatology than is reliance on medical prescriptions or interventive tactics—the latter often simply dampen or distort the way in which stress is felt rather than getting rid of it.

PART TWO

Defining and Locating
Your Problem

The next few chapters of *Coping with Your Grown Children* will help you to decide whether you, a midlife parent, actually do have a problem with your adult child. We will accomplish this by showing you how to analyze your family situation, and by then demonstrating how you may formulate and answer crucial questions about it. If your analysis reveals that a real problem exists, we will next help you decide whose problem it is. After all, it may be yours alone or it may be one you share with your child.

Once the problem is clearly outlined and responsibility for it definitively located, you will find yourself empowered to act on it directly rather than passively letting it act on you.

This and the next sections of the book will emphasize three problem-resolving principles:

- The absolute importance of establishing and maintaining good and open communications

- The fundamental value of using rational and systematic coping strategies

- The need to recognize and give first priority to individual rights and responsibilities—both your own and those of your child.

Observing these principles is imperative if you hope to deal at all effectively with the often wrenching problems you may at times confront with your adult offspring.

CHAPTER 4

WHOSE PROBLEM?
YOURS, MINE, OR OURS?

Dear Anne Landers:
I work as a flight attendant and am based in Chicago.
My mother lives in Kansas City. Whenever she sees
something in your column about smoking, drinking, doing dope,
or a single girl getting involved with a married man,
she clips it out and sends it to me.
I don't do any of this stuff and I wish she would stop treating
me like I was 12 years old. Maybe if you tell her she will listen.
Sign me—
Feet on the Ground

Introduction

Before attempting to solve a problem with your child, you, the middle-aged parent, need to work out the answers to several questions. They are fundamental, and will help you understand whether there is a problem (often there is not) and who owns the problem (is it your problem alone, your child's problem alone, or a shared problem?).

Simply put the questions are:

- What is <u>a</u> problem?
- What is <u>the</u> problem?
- What is the <u>real</u> problem?
- Whose problem is it?

Once the questions about the existence and ownership of problems are settled, we will describe procedures that you may wish to use in solving them, either unaided or with help.

Sometimes it may seem that nothing ever turns out quite right between parents and children, that problems and difficulties are the daily fare. In truth, though, the journey to adulthood usually occurs without undue hardship or upset for either children or parents. For most parents, children represent sources of satisfaction, delight, help, and amusement— and these feelings far outweigh the frustrations and exasperations that crop up as a normal part of the process of rearing them.

Though many families manage to avoid the more serious difficulties we are generally discussing here, there are millions who must still grapple with these painful situations— and the numbers are on the rise. This book is for these troubled families—and especially for the parents.

When Is There a Problem?

Isaiah is 38, hairy, heavily bearded, not known for his grooming or cleanliness. He has steered clear of gainful employment, living by getting money from his mother, who lives nearby. He is the only child. He makes some extra money out of various dubiously legal schemes. Once married, he left his wife and young son, apparently to enter into a series of short-lived liaisons with a succession of disagreeable women. He is rude, noisy, inconsiderate of others, and overbearing. He has no friends at all and his many detractors condemn him for his failure to abide by commonly accepted standards of cleanliness, honesty, self-reliance, and fidelity. That he mooches from his mother is especially hard for many to swallow.

The problem? In this instance there isn't one. Though Isaiah might represent a king-sized pain in another setting, his mother has both the resources and the wish to support him. His outspokenly boorish behavior, she believes, reflects his free, artistic spirit and she does not wish it to be bruised by having it rub against the abrasive environment so often found in the world of steady work. Isaiah, for his part, sees nothing wrong with what he is doing or has done; other people's opinions mean nothing to him. Since neither he nor his mother are troubled by the ordinary conventions, they are quite content with—and see nothing unusual about—their arrangement. It irks others who resent the flouting of the rules and the easy, irresponsible life it permits Isaiah to live. The problem, however, lies with the critics, not with Isaiah and his indulgent mama.

Certain conditions need to be met for a problem to exist between middle-aged parents and their adult children. There must be some situation (either real or imagined) and unfavorable (negative, disapproving, threatening) attitudes or opinions about that situation. The table below sketches it out.

Conditions Necessary for the Existence of a Problem

Attitudes or opinions about the situation	Situation	
	Imagined	Real
Favorable	No problem	No problem
Unfavorable	Problem	Problem

If a situation exists or is believed to exist, but the attitudes toward it are favorable (accepting, affirmative, or even neutral), there is no problem. A problem occurs only when some situation, either real or imaginary, gives rise to unfavorable (rejecting, disapproving, critical, resentful) attitudes.

"Feet on the Ground" (FOG), the flight attendant whose complaint appears at this chapter's opening, provides a good example of both kinds of problems. FOG's mother imagines that her daughter does, is capable of doing, or fears that she might do any of a variety of things of which she strongly disapproves. Even though the daughter is not guilty of any of these (in her mother's estimation) misbehaviors, the mother keeps sniping away at FOG.

The daughter is faced with a real situation in which the mother persists in insinuating—unfairly and wrongly—that FOG is misbehaving. She understandably and justifiably resents her mother's baseless innuendoes.

The two problems will disappear if:

- Mother realizes that her concerns are either unfounded and/or none of her business and stops her accusations; or if:

- Mother modifies her attitudes so that she accepts whatever situation may actually occur or that her busy imagination invents, and

- FOG learns to dismisss her mother's warnings and accusations.

In this instance, FOG's problem seems to be more pressing, but her indirect way of dealing with it is not especially promising, even if Mother happens to read the column carrying FOG's complaint. Mother's method of handling her problem is even more inappropriate and feeble.

What Is the Problem? (Finding the Problem)

In order to find a resolution to a troubling situation, the problem must first be correctly identified and accurately assigned to one or both of the parties involved. Sometimes the problem is quite apparent and requires very little analysis. If your son and daughter-in-law make a habit of unexpectedly dumping their two small children (your grandchildren) on you for protracted visits and this upsets you, you have an obvious problem. You know that you do not care for matters as they presently stand, and would like them to be different.

Other times it may not be quite so easy to sort things out. If you feel troubled or concerned about your relationship with your adult child, but cannot put your finger on what is causing these feelings, first try to state the problem clearly. Sit down in a quiet place and record as best you can the events that have disturbed you and the kinds of feelings that you have experienced. Suppose that your 23-year-old daughter, April, has been living with you for the past six months after graduating from college. She has a teaching credential, but no job. You and your husband, Jim, both work and are supporting April. The money isn't important, but you are beginning to feel troubled by April's continued presence. You write:

Date	Event (describe specifics)	Parent's feelings
11/2	April went out on an interview for a long-term substitute job. She wore jeans, T-shirt, leather jacket, jogging shoes. Her hair was straggly and she hadn't made up at all.	Angry, disappointed. I couldn't imagine going out on an interview looking like that. Sometimes I think she doesn't even want a job, the way she acts. I don't know what's the matter with her.
11/7	She didn't get up until 10 again this morning. Her clothes are strewn all over the house. When she got through showering she left three towels lying in a sodden heap.	I ask her to pick up and she does, but I hate having to be at her all the time. I wish she'd volunteer to do something on her own once in a while without being asked or told. I feel like a servant—her servant—around here.

(continued)

Date Event (describe specifics)	Parent's feelings
11/10 April borrowed my car to drive to the city for a concert. She didn't return until sometime the next day and she never called to say that she was staying over or that she was safely home.	I was worried sick. Jim had to drive me to work and that made him late—and angry. When I got home and saw the car in the driveway I was so relieved and furious at the same time. I was so mad I knew it wasn't the right time to speak up. I asked her if she'd had a good time and all she said was "Yeah." I went to my room and cried. That was all I could do.

And so on. When you have written down the events and your feelings, try to summarize what they mean to you, and *only* to you—not what they may mean *about* the child. Of April you might have said:

April's behavior disappoints, angers, and worries me. I am concerned that she has not found a job and gotten out on her own. I don't like having to continually remind her and ask her to help around the house and I wish she would be more considerate of Jim and me.

Be careful to state the problem entirely in your terms, limiting the statement to your feelings about whatever is happening. *Do not attribute qualities or motives to the child.* The kind of statement *not* to make might read:

April is lazy, ungrateful, inconsiderate, and selfish. Worst of all, she's uncaring, she doesn't give a damn for Jim and me or for our feelings.

Though all of these allegations may be true, none of them will help you with your problem and they won't help April with hers either. So, for openers, state the problem as it affects you.

What Is the Real Problem? (Consultation)

If you have misgivings about your diagnosis of the problem—and it pays to have your doubts early, rather than late, when the potential for lasting damage is greater—talk it over with someone you trust. The reason for this is simple—all too often there is a difference between the apparent and the real problem.

There may be difficulty in diagnosing the real problem because the apparent problem serves some other purpose—oftentimes an unconscious one, one not recognized or even suspected. An adult child may do something that both parents, deep down, feel neutral about. However, if the parents are not in a good place in their marriage, one or the other of them may seize on the child's behavior as a means of picking at the spouse without having to risk a direct assault. Consider this dialog:

> *"It's about time Sandy got out on her own."*
> *"I enjoy having her here. It's not that we can't afford it. Besides, with you gone so much of the time it makes me feel safer to have her here."*
> *"She's no better than a scrounger."*
> *"That's better than some of the things she could become. At least I know where she is. That's more than I can say for some people."*
> *"She should get out and start pulling her own weight, you know that. Why are you sticking up for her?"*

These parents are using the child's presence at home as a way of harassing one another without having to talk about *their* real difficulties. If Sandy did go away, matters would probably not improve; the parents would simply find another way of getting at one another.

Unearthing the real issue requires honesty, openness, and the willingness to let the chips fall where they may.

Because many of the things that we do are impelled by motives of which we are not at all, or only dimly, aware, consultation with another trusted person helps when a problem is being defined. This person can be a spouse, another child, a relative, a friend, a clergyman, a professional counselor. Tell this confidant the whole story as you see it and let him or her know what the problem seems to be, at least according to your lights. If it would prove embarrassing to have the matter become public knowledge, take care to select someone who can keep a confidence.

Once the background is traced and the problem laid out, ask your confidant whether he or she concurs with your statement of the problem. You will probably have to give more details before this can happen. When you receive the opinion, it may contradict your own diagnosis—but do not disregard it. Rather, restate the problem in terms acceptable to the consultant and then, if necessary, check out the restatement with a second confidant. This process will take time and effort, but it is necessary if you are to get to the heart of the matter.

Whose Problem Is It?

Once an adult child–parent problem is diagnosed, it must then be found to belong to one or more of the individuals involved. When there are only two possible parties—parents and child—the ownership possibilities are either mine (parents'), yours (child's), or, when the interests of both parties overlap, ours.

When there are more than two parties (persons or interests) involved (mother, stepfather, natural father, child, for example), the various perceptions of the problem and its possible location can become quite complicated. For the most part, we will limit our discussion to the two-party problem, in which the parents are considered a single entity. Nonetheless, the principles we will develop in this simplest case are extensible to any problem regardless of its complexity.

When adult children are concerned, problems most frequently occur because there is confusion or misunderstanding about precisely whose rights and responsibilities are involved. Children, when they become adults, naturally acquire certain rights, and their parents relinquish certain other responsibilities. Failure on the part of parents to relinquish those responsibilities that they can no longer legitimately claim makes for many difficulties. Charting out the rights and responsibilities of each party helps when it comes to locating the problem.

	Whose responsibility?	
Whose right?	Parent's	Child's
Parent's	Mine	Ours
Child's	Ours	Yours

If *both* the right and the responsibility belong to the parents, then the problem belongs to the parents—"Mine" in the table. If both belong to the child, then the problem is the child's, "Yours," and the parents should keep out of it.

When there is confusion about right and responsibility, then the problem is jointly owned, belonging both to parent and child ("Ours") and needing collective or collaborative action.

Getting rights and responsibilities straight is more easily said than done. Parents have resources, time, and ego invested in their children, and they will not normally give up either the child or their investments in them without a struggle. Above and beyond this, there is a time warp that often seems to afflict parents in which they see their offspring, not as they are now, but as children caught somewhere in the web of the past. By the same token, children often approach responsibility with understandable reluctance.

An adult child has the same rights and responsibilities as the parents do. These rights are spelled out in law and custom and include all the constitutionally guaranteed freedoms.

Responsibilities are also defined legally, as the parent of any teen-aged driver knows. The parent is "responsible" for the minor child; when children become adults they become "responsible" for themselves.

The failure of the child to take "responsibility" (or of the parent to relinquish it) may result in trade-offs.

"If you're going to live at home then we expect you to..."
"We'll support you while you're in college, but in return..."

If there are trade-offs—rights for responsibilities, or vice versa—a clear understanding about what right is being given up by the child and what responsibility is reverting to the parent is helpful.

A list of the rights and responsibilities of both parents and children would be wonderful to have, but these concepts are not absolute or universal, only matters of social or personal agreement. They depend on a host of considerations having to do with the values of both the individuals and the family. Thoughtful answers to the following questions may help the parent to sort matters out.

1. Do I have any responsibility for the behavior my child is exhibiting? Is it really any of my affair?
2. Does the child's behavior infringe on or limit any of my rights or freedoms?
3. Does the child have the right to behave that way, even though I may not like or accept it?

Honestly answering questions 1 and 2 "No" and the third "Yes" should signal you to keep from intervening in a particular instance. That's a "Your" (child's) problem.

If the opposite responses are made to any of these questions, then you (and possibly the child) do have a problem.

If you—the middle-aged parent—scrupulously attend to your own rights and responsibilities, and honor those of your troublesome offspring by maintaining a hands-off attitude, you should be able readily to decide whose problem some situation may be, regardless of the actions or circumstances that precipitated it.

Deciding on a Problem's Author or Authors

In addition to knowing who owns a problem, it helps to understand where it originated. Though the "no fault" concept might well save a great deal of grief if it could be successfully applied to intergenerational problems, that doesn't yet seem on the horizon, and given our refractory human natures, may never appear there.

Getting an idea of who is at fault (who has "authorship" of a problem, in my terminology) is important because it offers additional help in deciding how to deal with a problem. Essentially the same terms can be used to determine authorship as those used to fix ownership. Any specific problem may be "authored" by you, by me, or by us. When it is "us," that generally means there is only one problem. When it is "you" or "me," it may mean there are two problems, one growing from real, and the other from imaginary, roots.

The case of FOG and her mother illustrates the point. Each of them owns a problem whose author is clearly the mother and her imaginary fears. FOG has a real problem with her mother, but it is not the same one that mother has.

Andre and Marie have a married daughter, Celeste. Celeste came along late in the marriage and the parents were overjoyed because they had long believed that they would never be able to bring up a child of their own. They sacrificed to give Celeste everything they could. "Spoiled" as a young child, she has turned out to be an insensitive, self-centered, and demanding adult.

Celeste and her husband are expecting their first child and her parents are thrilled at the prospect. "How marvelous!" Marie exclaimed when she heard the news. "Celeste, dear, we want to do something. Let us buy the crib for the baby." Celeste and her husband had a decorator do the nursery and had the bill for over $2000 sent to Andre and Marie. They were thunderstruck. "What's this?" they wanted to know. "We said we'd buy the crib."

Celeste was furious. "You always do this," she ranted. "You always back away at the last minute, making commitments and not living up to them."

"But, honey, we didn't say the whole nursery," Marie tried to explain.

"Well, I certainly didn't understand it that way," Celeste snapped.

In this instance Celeste is clearly responsible—the author of this unhappy situation. She also has a problem that stems from her anger at what she regards as a broken promise. Andre and Marie have a real problem that will be worked out satisfactorily only in the unlikely event that Celeste admits that she is at fault for the misunderstanding and withdraws her demand. "Unlikely" states the prospect fairly because her parents have always caved in to her demands, so that she has no reason to give up on a winning combination. The parents do have some leverage, however—they don't have to pay the bill.

Any resolution that tilts to the parents' side will require them to resist to the point at which Celeste recognizes and admits to some fault. Then, when that happens, the parents might, if they chose, offer a compromise to soften the hurt and take the sting out of the admission. But, accepting fault is a difficult task; getting someone else to do it is even tougher.

By now you should have an idea about how to decide whether a problem exists, what it is, who has it, and who is mainly responsible for it. When this process is followed through and produces a result—a series of judgments—you are obliged to accept them unless fresh evidence shows that the analysis was clearly wrong. In short, once your conclusions are reached, stick with them.

Visualizing Solutions

Here are some suggestions about what you can do, specifically, to formulate solutions to problems. Often people are stumped because they simply do not see any possible actions they can take, do not know what to do or where to turn, and feel paralyzed by the circumstances. Of course, feeling this way may itself be a signal that you are ready to look for outside help. It is also a sign that serious, self-initiated action is needed right now. Some methods of generating possible solutions are presented in the following sections.

Self-Initiated Solutions

Let's assume that you confront a problem you do not want. Clearly you need to make changes. But how do you want things to be? Several techniques are available that will help you—the troubled parent grappling with a problem growing out of the relationship with an adult child—develop ideas for possible solutions. First, I will discuss real problems—those in which the parent has the right or the responsibility to intervene. Imaginary problems—those in which the parents wrongfully claim the right to be involved—will be covered later in this chapter.

For purposes of illustration, let's assume that your son, Emil, and daughter-in-law, Grace, have two children, Mark, four, and Ariel, who is going on three. They live nearby and the closeness makes it convenient for Grace to drop the children off while she goes shopping, gets her hair done, or runs other errands. It gradually dawns on you that the children are being left with you more and more often. Both of you enjoy the kids, but you alone, the grandmother, find yourself saddled with the responsibility of looking after the grandchildren because your husband is away at work most of the time. In addition to leaving the children more often, Grace has begun to do it without warning, dropping them off without clearing it with you first. You are fond of Grace, who is a good wife and mother and an attractive and ingratiating person. You do not want to offend her, so you have kept quiet about the inconvenience, even though you have had to give up activities of your own on several occasions. You are now growing resentful of the imposition and want to correct matters, but you cannot get up the nerve to act and you don't know exactly what to do.

The exercises sketched out below are designed to help overcome the experience of feeling conflicted, put upon, and helpless.

Fantasy

Sit back. Imagine what matters will be like next year if you do not do or say something now. What will matters be like *then?* Will Grace have suddenly stopped bringing the children around? Will she have decided to call ahead to see whether it will be convenient?

What will it be like in five years? Will there be more children by then? You will be getting older. Will you feel like caring for small children when you are five years farther along? Your husband will be retired by then. How will *he* take to this sort of imposition?

What about in ten years? The children will be older then. Will you want to have adolescents around? Taking care of preschoolers is one thing, but being in charge of older kids is altogether different.

What do you want your relationship with, and responsibility for, your grandchildren to be like? Do you enjoy having them? For how long? Do you mind caring for them? How often? What would it be like to say "No" to Grace or Emil if there is a conflict between your plan and theirs?

What about twenty years hence? How will it be to take on your great-grandchildren?

Why this fantasizing? Because it provides you with fresh perspectives and should lead to a clearer realization that unless you take action, matters will remain as they are. Recognizing that these problems do not ordinarily dry up and blow away—and that they can easily grow worse—is the first and most important step on the road to their resolution.

Projection

Though casting blame on others seldom helps (since it simply invites a reply in kind), an attempt to imagine why the children act as they do can serve as a springboard to well-considered and sensitive action on the part of the parents. Achieving understanding of the behavior of a child necessarily entails putting yourself in the child's shoes, so that you then view yourself, as nearly as you can manage it, from his or her standpoint. I call this process "projection."

"Why is Grace continually dropping the grandkids off?" you may ask. "What is it that allows her to think that this is perfectly all right?" So, you try to step into Grace's shoes for a time.

Most likely Grace imagines she is doing you a favor by bringing the grandchildren to stay with you. You say you like having them, they enjoy being with you, they like the cookies you always seem to have ready for them. That may well be it. Grace believes she is contributing to your sense of worth and value by dumping the kids off.

The failure to call in advance, what about that? Why can't she at least give word ahead of time? Well, maybe she thinks, "Poor Mom, she's at home alone most of the time, rattling around in that big house with nothing to occupy her. Having the children will be a nice treat for her. Give her something to do. Show her she's needed."

Both of these imaginary flights portray Grace in a positive light. She may be wrong or misguided (after all, who knows better than you that there's more to life than playing Granny), but she is acting out of honest concern for you—and she does trust the children with you.

Obviously it is important to put the most favorable interpretation possible on the child's actions. Starting from the premise that the child is uncaring, self-centered, or exploitative quickly leads to potentially wrong and destructive conclusions. Even when they *are* being terribly inconsiderate, most people fail to see their behavior in that light.

Assuming that the behavior of the adult child is founded in concern for the parents—or in benign ignorance of their feelings—is important simply because it is true most of the time. Coming to the painful conclusion that the child is acting out of hostility, cynicism, or blind selfishness makes effective action difficult although, unhappily, such motives sometimes do exist.

Informing Grace that you understand and appreciate her concerns at the same time that you request her to check with you in advance before leaving Mark and Ariel is much easier than simply telling her you disapprove of her practice and don't accept her rationale for it either.

Role Playing

Getting into another person's head is a tricky, and sometimes dangerous affair. The problem you hope to clarify may not open up to the projection technique—leaving you, for example, with no understanding of why it is that Grace is behaving as she does. You simply don't have a clue. When that occurs, getting someone to help you through the role-playing process is often revealing and productive.

To role-play you need a helper—perhaps the confidant you talked with earlier—to serve as counterfoil. The process is not unlike playing "house" or "school" as a child. Perhaps you will have your friend portray you, and you will become Grace, for purposes of the drama. Set the stage so that it reflects the real-life situation.

Let it be, say, a Thursday morning when Grace bounces in unannounced, full of smiles, Mark and Ariel in tow. She is on her way to have her hair and nails done. You have just returned from shopping, hot and tired. You had planned to have a bath and a quiet lunch and then a nap.

Setting the situation in this way, you and your partner then act it out. It could lead anywhere, but it is important that the actors in the drama do their level best to reveal true feelings and not to put forth the polite, socially acceptable, dishonest chatter that has been the common fare in this troublesome situation up until now. Properly done, this plain-speaking will get a handle on what you and Grace have really been thinking and saying (and on what you ought to, or might otherwise, be thinking and saying) and thus open the way for productive and mutually acceptable corrective measures.

As we have seen, then, the techniques of fantasizing, projecting, and role-playing can each help to clarify a problem and encourage doing something about it. Once this need for action is understood and accepted, the next step is to sort out the kinds of strategies that might work and the consequences, positive and negative, that can be associated with each such approach. We will review this latter process in Chapter 18.

Handling Imaginary Problems

Real problems, such as the simple one discussed above, are relatively easy to address and resolve. But what of imaginary ones—those problems that middle-aged parents and their adult children concoct or invent, and that so complicate their relationships with one another? What can be done to bring these problems out into the open, where they can be seen and addressed?

This is a much more difficult matter because self-initiated procedures for elucidating a problem and formulating various solutions are not likely to pan out. The best approach that parents can take is to be honest and open about their feelings, and to try to express them in such a way that they can be received calmly and constructively.

To see that a problem is an imaginary one—your imaginary one, more likely than not—outside help may be needed. Sometimes, as with the methods of finding the real problem, a confidant will assist greatly. Role-playing is especially useful in revealing that the plight, as we imagine it, does not exist. But, when the puzzle is complex, or one that grows out of baseless fear or dread, then working with other people can help immeasurably.

Aided Solutions

Problems that involve adult children and their parents cannot help but block all participants from realizing the full measure of satisfaction and fulfilment from what ought to be a mature relationship among all parties. Indeed, sometimes the participants in the problem do not fully appreciate that it exists. Can the mother who cheerfully, unfailingly, and unquestioningly accepts exploitation and domination by her children be said to have a problem? Folk wisdom would counsel "If it ain't broke, don't fix it." And indeed, there is no point in unearthing such problems if bringing them into the light will only result in resentment, acrimony, and misery all around. However, when unhappiness, resentment, or hostility already exist, clarification—to the extent that some reasonable course of action can be settled on—seems a logical step. The various sources of help, and advice on how best to use them, are provided in Chapter 20.

Groups

The heightened realization that individuals sharing similar problems can be an important source of aid to one another has led to the emergence of a large variety of groups designed to achieve new understandings and to find new ways of dealing with problems of every kind.

This so-called Human Potential Movement takes many different forms, some of which are: Gestalt, Transactional Analysis (TA), Self-Awareness, T-groups, Human Relations Workshops, Sensitivity Training, Encounter Groups, Support Groups, etc. They address their attention to many goals—raising consciousness, increasing sensitivity or assertiveness, promoting personal growth, offering psychotherapy, providing the opportunity to share, to learn, and to change.

These groups draw different kinds of individuals together: men, women, parents, single parents, gays, parents of gays, alcoholics, handicapped, parents of handicapped, seniors, couples, and so on. Almost any sizable community will offer group experiences through churches, community organizations, extension or evening divisions of the local college or university, adult education programs, YMCA, YWCA, and many other facilities. Some discussion groups exist for purposes of sharing and growth; others are designed to address specific problems, such as mid-life crises, lack of assertiveness (a quality commonly observed in the relationship between middle-aged parents and their children), bearing up under loss or personal disaster, and so on.

The primary purpose of such a group is to provide the member a different perspective on one's own self through the feedback received from others. The impressions that others have of us and of our problems, whether real or imagined, can be a source of especially useful insights.

Finding an appropriate group entails getting in touch with the various organizations or agencies that sponsor them. A call to any of the groups mentioned above should turn up the opportunities available. When these groups are located, one should talk to the local leader first to find out the specific purpose or goal of the group and any other information you need to know—fees, for example, which are sometimes nominal, and which are sometimes exorbitant. At that time, you should also find out about the time, place, and duration of the group's meetings and any special requirements they may have. Sometimes there may be a retreat for a weekend, for example, and it helps to know, in advance, about any special demands that may be put on you.

The qualifications and training of the group leader who will be presiding over and guiding your activity must also be verified. In particular, you should check the academic background and experience the leader has had with other programs in the past. Steer clear of groups led by untrained or inexperienced persons. A Master's degree in psychology or a related human services field, plus certification in the form of a state license or credential, ought to be the minimally acceptable qualification.

Among the various kinds of support groups, you should also know of Toughlove. Toughlove originally evolved as an approach to dealing with rebellious, troublesome teenagers, primarily runaways or substance abusers. Although these kinds of problems are still its main focus, the movement also strives to offer help and backing to parents attempting to deal with older kids who present parents the kinds of difficulties discussed here.

Toughlove's program is based on a set of ten beliefs that participants in the parent/community support groups must work to understand and accept. Perhaps its most prominent features are the recognition that children and parents both need to observe limits in what they can, or are allowed to, do. The support groups work to enable parents—and to assist actively where this is necessary—to establish these limits.

Toughlove also aims at restructuring parents' attitudes toward themselves and their children, helping them to become more realistic about and more aware of their children's behavior. It is a tough-minded, realistic approach that would seem to be useful in dealing with outspokenly intransigent behavior. It also offers an approach to learning to live with the problem (if the problem itself cannot be managed) that might be useful to many distraught parents.

PART THREE

Shared Problems of Parents and Adult Children

Up to this point, we have learned how to decide whether there is a problem between parents and their grown children and, if so, whose problem it is.

This next few chapters will discuss the nature of several specific issues that cause tension between the generations, illustrating them in detail, and offering suggestions for their resolution. The syndromes we will now consider are:

- The Unemptied Nest (children who do not leave home)
- "Uncut Cords" or "Stay-at-Homes"
- Dangling Grandchildren
- Fall Shorts (children who do not live up to their potential)
- Meddlesome Grandparents (the three-generation dilemma)
- Injury and Illness
- Stepparents and Stepchildren
- Legal, Fiscal, and Other Scrapes

In the great majority of instances, these syndromes are likely to be examples of "Our" problems—ones shared by both parent and child. Depending on circumstances, however, they can occasionally amount to individual difficulties for either the parent ("Mine") or the child ("Yours"). For the specific problems presented and analyzed in Chapters 5–11, this individual placement is very much the exception.

My hope in undertaking a discussion of these tribulations is that there will be a threefold result: First, that you, the middle-aged parent, will realize that problems such as these are much more common than you might have believed and that you are not alone in your plight; that there are causes or explanations for them that exist outside the parent–child relationship; and, third and most important, that specific actions can be taken to meet and deal with them systematically, positively, and constructively.

CHAPTER 5

THE UNEMPTIED NEST

You can't go home again—or can you?

Introduction

Most counselors have known for some time now that there is a growing problem with children who never leave home or who, having left it, return, seemingly for good.

In this chapter, I will offer some examples, drawn from my experiences as a counselor, of what I call the Unemptied Nest. Naturally, in these and all other illustrations or examples throughout the book, the names of the counselees and many other details have been changed in order to protect the privacy of the persons concerned.

I hadn't seen Ralph in years. Once we lived in the same neighborhood, and his kids and ours had gone to elementary school together. When we chanced on one another not long ago, he didn't even stop to say hello. "I've got a problem. Can you help me with a problem?" he blurted.

"Let's go someplace where we can talk," I suggested. We went to a nearby cafeteria, found our way to a quiet table at the back. "Tell me about it," I said. His story tumbled out, full of anger, frustration, guilt, and disappointment.

Ralph, a high-ranking civil servant, lived in a comfortable home in a good, suburban neighborhood. Alice, his wife, also worked full-time as a secretary. His anger centered around his son, Steve, the youngest of three children. Steve had lived at home while attending college. He had graduated with good grades and a major in economics four years earlier. Upon graduating he had looked for a job for a while, but when initially unsuccessful, had gradually given up searching. He kept on living at home, where his presence was a constant, minor irritant to Ralph.

Steve's being at home was bad enough, although Ralph and Alice had worked out a way of coping with that situation, essentially by making believe that it did not exist. Even after four years they nourished the belief that Steve would be getting out any day now. Then, a few days before Ralph ran into me, their older son, Mike, lost his job. He, too, came back home.

Ralph simply couldn't handle both of these adult male children being there more or less permanently. They weren't supposed to be home; they were supposed to be out making their own way in the world. They weren't supposed to be dependent on their parents. They weren't supposed to be lounging around the family room when he and Alice returned home from work. They weren't supposed to be draining off his and Alice's time, energy, and resources while doing nothing around the house, giving nothing in return. But they were, and Ralph was uncomprehending, furious, and helpless, all at the same time.

That coffee break lasted over two hours. By the time it ended we had managed to accomplish three things.

First, Ralph had unloaded a great deal of his anger and frustration. He had talked about his problems and his feelings about them, and he felt better for it.

Second, he heard from me that his problem was not all that uncommon and that he should stop accepting blame for whatever it was that had gone wrong.

Third, he learned that he could do something about the situation, that he was not helpless after all.

Talking about his feelings gave temporary relief, though the other things that happened during our talk were more important and led, eventually, to the discovery that his wife and children fully shared his own feelings of helplessness and desperation. This brought them all to a point of common understanding that allowed them to begin to deal with their shared problem directly, rationally, and constructively.

This process did not run its course easily or all at once. It began with an intensely emotional discussion between Ralph and Alice during which they both came to understand that indeed they had a problem. They then sat down with their sons to express, forthrightly, their own concerns. This tense session revealed that the boys, in their own ways, were just as troubled as the parents. The parents and boys then mutually decided it would be best to seek outside help. They began to meet regularly with a family counselor, who eventually steered Steve and Mike into a career planning program being offered through the university in town. All this took much time and some money, but a year after that first encounter Ralph was able to report that the boys had found work—not great jobs, true, but ones that gave them some satisfaction, held reasonable promise, and provided a living. Steve was still staying home, then, but was now contributing to its upkeep and thinking of moving out on his own, a prospect that made Ralph jubilant.

Ralph's experience neatly illustrates a number of points that will be returned to repeatedly throughout the book. This problem cropped up in spite of Ralph's and Alice's conscientious and well-intentioned efforts. It developed because of their failure to bring the issue out in the open for discussion. It grew, slowly and insidiously, to the point that it caused severe conflict and posed a real threat to the health and well-being of the entire family. And, happily, it was resolved satisfactorily through forthright and logical action and a courageous willingness to admit the need for and to actively seek outside help.

How It Used To Be

Of the scores of boys and young men I grew up with, only two of them did not get away from home at the very first opportunity—both were disabled. Most young men moved out just as soon as they found a job that paid them enough to support themselves. With the young women I knew, the pattern was a bit different. They might work and live at home for a time, but as soon as they could they married and went off to set up housekeeping. If marriage did not happen, they too left home. Any normal young person of my generation and socio-economic–ethnic group wished to and did get away from home, for keeps, as soon as he or she was able.

It is not quite like that any more, even though most children eventually do leave home. Many do not, though, or take their good old time about it. Parents have a good deal of difficulty understanding and coping with this new pattern of behavior when it occurs.

Why Adult Children Do Not Leave Home

People now in their fifties almost invariably struck out on their own to achieve a measure of the privacy, self-sufficiency, and self-determination that they were so frequently denied at home. In earlier times, homes were usually smaller than they are now, bedrooms were often shared, and doors remained open because God only knew what the children would get up to when left to their own devices. A house had a bathroom—singular—and a rigid set of priorities for its use. Children did not have priority, except over younger children. With very little privacy, continual reminders of dependency, and limited freedom, children cried out to abandon their parent's confining homes.

In the last half century things have changed. First, the attitudes of parents toward children have undergone a transformation. Our whole society has become more permissive, learning to treat them as individuals with rights, needs, and problems of their own. Children now routinely receive or earn allowances and, as they get older, begin collecting other perks. Their own rooms. Perhaps a private telephone. An automobile. Charge accounts.

This shower of good things became possible because the material conditions of life improved for much of the population. People, especially those in the white middle-class, enjoyed a significant enhancement of their standard of living. Pay went up faster than prices, credit became easier, jobs were readily available, disposable income shot up.

The increased resources made housing accessible that provided every member of the family (excepting mother) with his or her own space.

In addition to more comfortable, private, and convenient living accommodations—accommodations that did not actively encourage the children to parachute from an overcrowded nest—other changes were happening that tended to prolong the dependency of the child. The average educational level increased to the point where a majority of high school graduates at least started college.

Since 1970 the rising level of education has been accompanied by an equally sharp decline in the availability of jobs requiring post-secondary training. During the 50s and 60s, college-trained persons, especially males, encountered little difficulty in finding work commensurate with their training. Good jobs were plentiful and college-trained applicants were in short supply.

This all changed. Graduates began to experience trouble finding work that had any direct bearing on, or relevance to, their training. This discrepancy between expectation and reality frustrated and discouraged many. Some returned home disappointed, unwilling or unable to work at jobs for which their education had either not prepared or overprepared them. It was not a matter of them not wanting work so much as the right kind of work not wanting them.

For the person not trained in college, matters were by no means easier. Unemployment rates for young people have consistently run two to three times above the national average and for certain groups it has been even higher than that.

Oftentimes the work, when there was any available, was part-time or paid so little that the net take home pay would not support the person trying to make it alone, independently. So they basically fell to living at home until things improved.

The inability to find appropriate work has not been as catastrophic a burden as it once might have been because the parents often were able to support the child, to help out, to tide him or her over. And, as the individual quest for work wore on and eventually, wore out, what had been thought of as a temporary arrangement imperceptibly became a permanent one. The parents could still afford it. After all, both of them had jobs.

There was another force at work, too. Though marriage might be deferred, the institution itself was proving fragile. People married later, but the marriages often proved short-lived. When the marital breakup came, one or sometimes both of the partners would seek haven with parents. Even though divorce is commonplace and no longer carries the social stigma it once did, a failed marriage still levies heavy personal costs and may immobilize its victims for a substantial period of time—enough time to make the process of getting established difficult and anxiety-producing.

Less obviously, underlying social and cultural changes have made it more costly to rear children. To provide space, to enhance opportunities, to ensure a measure of independence, privacy, and freedom all take money. Parents know this. The "middle-class poor" are a recent phenomenon and parents in that group understandably look forward to the day when their children will be gone and they themselves can begin to enjoysome of the resources previously devoted to the children. This may dispose the parents, consciously or unconsciously, to push and the children may push right back, refusing to cooperate by taking the first big step out of the nest. Sometimes it almost seems as if the children are trying to make things difficult, awkward, or uncomfortable for the old folks.

So, a variety of forces are at work in keeping children from leaving home. The ones mentioned here are:

- Sheer comfort and convenience
- Increasing average age at marriage
- A rising divorce rate
- An increasing average educational level
- A decline in employment opportunities, especially for the young
- Reaction by children against parental eagerness to have the children out on their own

Any one or a combination of these factors may prevent a child from leaving home. This does not necessarily make for a problem, however. If the parents do not mind, of if they actually prefer to have the child at home, no harm is done. If the presence of the child in the home past the expected time of departure actually does lead to strife of one sort or another—to open conflict, to feelings, on either side, of hostility, anger, frustration, and despair—then the situation calls out for correction.

Blaming and Fault Finding

The temptation to fix responsibility or blame needs to be avoided in the case of the child with the uncut cord. The reason? It is usually impossible to lay fault at a single door.

Linda, 24, an only child, has everything—looks, clothes, a degree, a Porsche. The father, Ed, complained to me about Linda. "She's just running around, having a good time. She has her degree, but she hasn't made a move about getting a job. Been doing that for two years now."

"And you want her to be out on her own?"

Ed looked at me pityingly. "Of course, Beth and I won't be able to take care of her forever."

"Tell me about her situation."

Linda lived rent-free in a mother-in-law cottage behind the family home. Everything in it was supplied by her parents, who also gave her unlimited use of their credit cards and a generous monthly allowance. What had prompted Ed's concern was the insurance bill on the Porsche—Linda's driving habits had landed her in an assigned risk pool.

"Ed, do you think that maybe Linda has no reason to get up and out?" I asked. "You're giving her the kind of life that would be the envy of anybody. Wouldn't you like to be in her shoes?"

Ed reflected about it for a moment. "Well, maybe. Except I thought people naturally wanted work, wanted to be free, on their own."

"Linda is on her own, more on her own than anyone who works and gets told what to do part of the day. She has it all and she doesn't have to give up anything for it."

Ed went on to talk of independence and self-respect, but finally wound up acknowledging that Linda had a good deal and he couldn't blame her for holding on to it.

"Have you ever discussed her getting out on her own?"

The matter had never been brought up. Ed and Beth complained to one another, but they had never broached the subject to Linda.

"What do you want to happen?"

"I guess I'd like her to be on her own. Able to look after herself without me and Beth helping," Ed replied.

"How does Beth feel about it?"

"I guess I don't really know."

In this case it is easy for those who identify with the parents to see Linda as inconsiderate, selfish, and spoiled, one who has totally failed to learn the value of work and self-reliance. It is equally easy to point the finger of blame at the parents by noting that they hadn't even bothered to talk about their needs and feelings to one another, much less to Linda.

Situations such as this develop gradually and it takes time to unravel them. Once Ed saw the glaring need to talk the matter out, he acted on it—not angrily or impulsively, but in an open, nonblaming way. He learned that Beth was not quite so eager to have Linda leave as he was because she feared that without the slight amount of oversight and guidance that she and Ed were able to provide, Linda might get into some kind of unimagined, vague "trouble." Beth had very little confidence in Linda's ability to take charge of her own life and that was one underlying reason for the prolonged dependency relationship. Linda was still a little child in Beth's eyes.

Linda had fewer qualms. She disclosed that she was growing bored with the life she was leading and had wanted to find something to do. She began looking seriously and, through a friend, found a job in an advertising agency. She discovered that she was good at the work, she learned quickly, and she was promoted to account executive in a short time. She soon left the mother-in-law cottage and managed on her own—not well at first, but adequately.

Linda's case illustrates a situation in which the home is so comfortable that there is simply no physical or economic reason to leave it. She was just doing what comes naturally and she was helped in this by parents who, in some ways, did not want her to go, not believing that she had the ability to fend for herself. Moreover, her parents had had neither the courage nor the common sense to talk with her openly about feelings they were concealing from her. Fortunately, when they got to the point at which they could bring these things into the open, there was sufficient care for one another and sufficient agreement about both the nature of the problem and of the desirable solutions for it that the matter could be resolved comfortably and constructively.

How to Build a Permanent Dependent

Not every cord-cutting effort succeeds.

When Chris and Martha divorced after 25 years of marriage, Chris gained custody of their youngest child, Grant. The breakup was extremely bitter and Chris regarded getting custody of Grant as a victory over Martha. He lavished care and attention on Grant, trying to anticipate all his needs, satisfy all his whims. He continued to treat Grant like a 10-year-old even when Grant was 21 and larger than his strapping father. The last thing Chris wanted was to offend his son and drive him back to his mother.

Chris did try to ease Grant out on his own by giving him a time limit to find a job and move out. However, when the deadline arrived, Grant had made no move and Chris let it go by unnoted.

A series of ultimatums came and went, each unheeded. Finally the matter was resolved after a fashion by Chris' decision to remarry and move out of the apartment he and Grant had shared. His new arrangement made no provision for

Grant, who was forced, finally, to be responsible for himself. This went badly because Grant couldn't find work. He couldn't even manage to look for it because he dreaded approaching potential employers. Now in psychotherapy, he scrapes along on handouts from his mother, with whom he has been staying. Chris is sorry about Grant's plight, but blames it all on Martha.

Working Out a Solution

When coping with the child who has not left home—or has found the way back there—it will help you to keep these things in mind:

- You need to gain the full participation of everyone concerned.
- Establish an atmosphere for discussion that is fair-minded, open, constructive, and as free from acrimony, anger, and guilt-laying as you can make it.
- Work to unearth the real problem. (In the case of the un-emptied nest, the continued presence of the child sometimes enables the parents to get at one another without dealing with the underlying issue, usually an unhappy or strife-torn marriage.)
- Remember that being 21 or older does not necessarily qualify a child to go it alone. Protected by their parents, many children have hadno opportunity to learn survival skills; most pick them up readily enough when they must, but knowing how to locate and land a job or a place to live or how to do the laundry or prepare a meal are complex tasks, ego-threatening when faced, ego-shattering when failed. The prospect of defeat may be sufficiently intimidating to immobilize the child. When this happens, outside help may be necessary.

With all of these cautions and grim warnings, it may appear as though getting the child out of the nest calls for consummate diplomatic and psychological skills. That is not necessarily so, although it is not quite so simple as the suggestion often put forward by individuals who have not had to live through the complicated and wrenching difficulty of dealing with an adult child still at home. They blithely dismiss the problem. "What's so hard about that?" they are likely to demand. "Kick the kid out!"

In one way they are right. Tossing the child out will solve one problem. The trouble with that solution is that it might unloose a flood of difficulties even more painful than than the original one had been. It should be obvious that dropping the eviction bomb will affect the feelings and interrelationships of everyone touched by the decision. Relations might get better (unlikely, but possible), stay about the same, or worsen, at least for a time and perhaps permanently.

The process of coping with the problem of the Unemptied Nest—the decisions, alternatives, and consequences of each—is worked out in detail in Chapter 19. There we illustrate the Decision Tree method of resolving problems rationally and with as little pain as possible. This procedure should be studied carefully if you are troubled with a stay-at-home child.

When Not to Push

Feathered fledglings are shoved out of the nest for one of two reasons: either the parents sense that the young are ready to fly off on their own or they determine in some inexplicable way that it has little or no chance of survival and its continued presence would threaten the rest of the brood.

The concept of readiness is crucial when it comes to the human nestling. If there is reason to believe that the time is not right, the appropriate tactic is to try to find out more clearly just why the child is not ready and to correct whatever it is that is holding him or her back.

The state of readiness varies from individual to individual. Some are ready to take off and manage on their own when extremely young; others mature more slowly or find themselves in situations where a long period of dependence seems built in. Judge a child's readiness for independence by keeping your eyes open and by talking to the child and others who know her or him well and thus are able to offer informed and objective opinions. When required, call in outside help to promote changes in outlook and in the situation itself. Birds always learn to fly after being thrust out of the nest, but the analogous approach is not always appropriate for our human offspring.

Getting Help

Urging the adult child to move out may bring the discovery that the problem is more severe and deep-seated than you can manage, and thus force you to acknowledge that some sort of outside help is necessary.

Depending on the situation and the individuals involved, the specific kind of help required will vary from one instance to another. The method outlined in Chapter 20 will help you sort through and identify just what kind of problem you have and search out that help most appropriate to the situation.

One common characteristic of stay-at-homes is that there are problems in seeking and securing work. This often represents a touchy state of affairs for a number of reasons. The parents may place what seems to be an excessive value on work (and its implied autonomy) so far as the children are concerned. Repeated past failures at finding work may well discourage or even immobilize the child. Not knowing where or how to start looking, coupled to continual nonconstructive nagging from the parents, can produce the same effects. Disagreements about where, how, or at what level of employment to start also contribute to the climate of tension and conflict.

There are many resources and strategies that have been successfully followed in finding appropriate work. They do vary considerably in their success, depending on just how compatible an individual's skills, training, interest, and capabilities may be with the job for which he or she has launched a search. This broad field has been surveyed and analyzed by Richard Bolles, whose *What Color Is Your Parachute?* fully lives up to the promise carried in its subtitle—"A Practical Manual for Job Hunters and Career Changers."

The procedures and analyses advocated by Bolles are relevant and useful, and their effectiveness can be materially improved if a number of job hunters work through the exercise together. Observing the problems and quandaries, and learning of the successes and failures of others, does a great deal to motivate and reassure the seeker. Many career counseling services—especially university or college placement bureaus or extension divisions, as well as some private or public placement organizations—are providing exactly such experiences in addition to offering help with resumé preparation, interview opportunities, job canvassing strategies, and the like. Though a fee may be involved, the experience, the information to be gained, and the possible favorable consequences justify the outlay here. As in any other relationship with a source of help, be sure that you first ascertain the qualifications of the individual or institution offering the service.

Finally, the parent may want to know how best to behave during the period of active job search. This, too, is a difficult assignment because so much rides on it for both child and parent. Being helpful, interested, constructive, and supportive without displaying either excessive anxiety or the sort of nitpicking interest that will annoy or turn the job-seeker off is probably best in most such situations. If the child's search is energetic and persistent, the goals reasonable, and the desire to work authentic, something will ultimately turn up.

Chapter 6

DANGLING GRANDCHILDREN

Happiness is being a grandparent.

Introduction

One of the great things about having grandchildren, most grandparents would agree, is that you have them only in small doses. After a few hours their parents pack them back home until the next visit. Grandparents have all the fun of indulging the children without the associated burden of work and responsibility. Not always, though.

Robin is 30. She and her husband were divorced two years ago.

She had been working full-time when the split occurred. She kept on with her job, but she was badly unsettled by the experience and moved back home with her parents. She has custody of the children and they came with her—Kelly, now four, and Kim, six years old.

The grandparents are in their late fifties. At first they were glad to help out, but they are beginning to tire of the work, the cost, and the responsibility. Added to this is the fact that Robin has recently been able to pick up the pieces of her life and has resumed dating. On a few recent occasions she has stayed away all night, and the parents disapprove of this development strongly.

Robin, for her part, appreciates what her parents have done, although their veiled criticisms of her recent behavior trouble her. She would like to be more on her own, with the children, but she has no resources to move out. Her former husband has never contributed to the support of the children and dropped out of sight soon after the dissolution. She is hesitant about taking the children out of their stable, secure, and loving environment.

Being faced with the unexpected and unwelcome task of bringing up small children when there was every reason to believe that this onerous chore was firmly behind them is one of the newer problems facing middle-aged parents. The incidence of such situations is on the increase, partly because of the climbing divorce rate, but other factors also contribute. The willingness of the courts to award custody to the male parent adds complications that often draw in the grandparents, as does the growing tendency for unmarried women to bear and to raise a child. In these instances, the single parent who works needs help with the care of the child and the duty often falls to the grandparents—especially the grandmother.

Another source of distress that arises when separations occur is that the children often accompany one of the parents to a distant location. This development has the effect of denying at least one set of grandparents the privilege—and some would call it a right—of enjoying regular contact with their grandchildren.

Although most grandparents will step in to help in an emergency out of a sense of family obligation, when the situation becomes protracted they may grow alienated because of the accompanying sense of helplessness, of having no alternative. This feeling of impotence and loss of control undermines the self-perception of order and competence most of us need and value in our lives, something the grandparents thought they had won permanently once their child left.

In other, earlier days the family was more extended in form. Then, the physical or temporal separation of its members was not so great. There were more hands available to share the work and the responsibility of caring for a small child so that the attitudes about receiving and looking after it were more accepting and easygoing. Under those conditions a supportive, nurturing environment could readily be provided. But with the downsizing and restructuring of the family, the sudden introduction of a small new member who upsets the well-ordered routine and imposes an onerous and unsought responsibility does not make for the best or most wholesome atmosphere in which to bring up that child.

Resolving the Responsibility Question

Often middle-aged parents left with the care of grandchildren are hamstrung because of their reluctance to declare their own freedom. Their children saddle them with the grandchildren either because they are imperfectly aware of the weight of the burden they are imposing, because they know what it is but don't know what else to do, or (rarely) because they simply don't give a damn.

When the behavior of the adult children is predicated on a misunderstanding or on an underestimation of the weight of the load being heaped on the shoulders of the grandparents, the obvious response is to inform the adult child just what is involved in terms of extra work and cost to you, and to communicate openly the feelings that accompany this sudden increase in your responsibilities.

A number of components contribute to the dimensions of this extra burden of care, including: a definite and recordable number of hours of work; the outlay of resources for transportation, food, clothing, and medical or dental treatment; a portion of the ordinary expenses of maintaining and operating the household—heat, light, water, gas, rent, and so on. All of these can be recorded and reckoned in such a way as to give the parents a fair idea of what keeping the child demands of the grandparents in terms of additional time, effort, and money.

It makes equal good sense to inventory and report your own feelings to your grown child. Do you really want responsibility for the care of the child? Are you willing to accept it on a long-term basis? Do you prefer another arrangement? What level of assistance would you be comfortable with providing? What precisely are you willing to do? What extra burdens does having care of the child place on you and your partner physically, psychologically, and socially?

Analyzing the situation and setting down all its personal, fiscal, and social costs and benefits should enable you, the grandparents, to define the conditions under which you are willing and able to help—if indeed you are. If you are not up to the responsibility, you should say so, giving your reasons.

Since the problem of Dangling Grandchildren is studded with a host of conflicting feelings, needs, and pressures, resolving it calls for discretion. Though you may not want what you've been stuck with, the child's parent is likely not in a good place either. He or she may not want you troubled with the care of the child, either out of concern for you or the child, but has no other place to turn. Money problems may enter in, and there may also be disagreement between you and the child's parent about the nature, frequency, and severity of discipline. This latter disagreement may well affect the child, who has to reconcile conflicting sets of rules or signals.

Sherm has a 7-year-old son, Tad, by a previous marriage. He and his present wife, Edie, both work and leave the boy with Sherm's mother, Paula. Paula is very strict with Tad, paddling him when he acts up, washing his mouth out with soap when he speaks what she terms "filth," keeping him from playing with other children. Paula is glad to look after Tad because she believes it "keeps her young" and because she is obsessed with the idea of duty and obligation to family. Edie and Sherm are much more easy-going, openly affectionate, and tolerant of Tad than Paula is. Tad is confused by the continually shifting rules and came to my attention when the parents brought him in to discuss his sudden, violent, uncontrollable temper tantrums. He had also begun having frequent, severe headaches. As we explored the situation the conflicting periods of harsh and relaxed discipline seemed to be implicated. Accordingly, Tad was enrolled in an extended daycare program at his school. His behavior improved dramatically and his headaches stopped.

Paula had great difficulty accepting her displacement, however, and now feels as if she has not only failed, but been rejected. Efforts to explain the problem have not helped to dispel her feelings of inadequacy and diminished worth.

When the child's parent neither considers nor cares about the effects on the grandparents, there is no basis on which a workable compromise can be reached. This is a difficult situation for the grandparents to find themselves in, and they are likely to have few options, all of them troubling. When faced with this situation, grandparents need to keep in mind that *they are no longer responsible for the actions of their adult children.* Though they may feel a sense of obligation, that sense is not a commandment.

They had little or no part in the chain of events that have led up to the existing situation. It was not their decision to contract the marriage, to beget children, to do any of the things that have contributed to what is being treated as a shared problem.

They do have recourses or options. When minor children are involved, parents cannot simply turn off responsibility like a faucet. It can be given up or taken away, but only after formal legal steps are taken. Invoking legal remedies to correct a situation involving grandchildren is a distasteful, last-ditch alternative, but they are there and those available can be found by consulting one's private attorney, the public prosecutor, the juvenile authorities, or such independent agencies as Children's Aid. The drawback in taking legal steps is that they solve some problems at the often considerable risk of creating others that are worse, so they are generally a last resort. When necessary, however, parents can be ordered to take full custody, pay support, or, when unable or unwilling to provide these, to relinquish responsibility for their offspring.

The other difficulty—the loss of contact with grandchildren because of geographical or other considerations—is sometimes a knotty dilemma. If you, the grandparents, find it difficult to accept the separation, then your obvious tack is to communicate your concerns and desires, and to propose a solution. The options available depend on the distances involved and the resources at hand, but could take a variety of forms—regular phone calls, periodic visits (there or here, with some sort of agreement about travel costs if the children come to you), summer vacation stays, and the like. To arrive at a tolerable compromise, it is important to keep in mind that the child and the child's custodian have their own feelings and commitments, and that these will often rule out a solution that would be ideal from your standpoint. To help in understanding and anticipating some of these hurdles, role-playing (as described in Chapter 4) may be especially fruitful.

Getting Help

Where Dangling Grandchildren are involved, a number of different issues may surface, each of which will require aid from a different outside source of assistance. With intrapersonal or interpersonal conflicts, any of the various kinds of individual or group help resources described in Chapter 20 may be appropriate and useful. Because the fallout from this dilemma may prove particularly widespread, affecting child, parent, and grandparent, family counseling is often an especially appropriate resource.

When the thorny questions of support and custody are involved, the local Family Service Agency (often a privately supported organization providing various kinds of specialized assistance to troubled families) is a useful starting point. It is listed in the white pages of the telephone directory.

Government organizations—local Welfare, federal Social Security—furnish aid when certain categories of need are present. Child care, especially extended daycare, is increasingly available through schools or school-like arrangements at minimal or no cost to users. Grandparents do not need to take on the whole burden of care.

If legal issues or questions are present, the Legal Aid Society (also a telephone directory, white-page number) can point one toward various sources of legal counsel.

CHAPTER 7

FALL SHORTS

Lucien's mother...began to tell Lucien she was disappointed in him....From then on, this disappointment would be her principal theme. "You are the leading killjoy of my life," she assured him. "God will pay you back for disappointing me."

Introduction

"Fall Shorts" doesn't refer to something you pull on after Labor Day. It is a term for children who do not live up to their potential—"underachievers." These are talented children, or so we believe, who somehow do not perform at a sufficiently high economic and status level, or do not attain some high goal of the parents, thus proving a grave disappointment to themselves and/or their parents. This common problem, similar to and even, in many instances, coterminous with that of the Unemptied Nest (*see* Chapter 5) can be a knotty one. Middle-aged parents, especially, are prone to believe that America is a land of unlimited opportunity in which each person determines his or her own success. We imagine that anyone, given the right combination of talent, luck, and application, can aspire to anything.

Dave, a very hard-working and extremely successful businessman, came from a blue-collar background. He was the first in his family to go to college, where he did well. He and his wife, Madge, have three children. The youngest, Duane, is the problem. Duane graduated from high school in the upper third of his class. His counselor told Dave that Duane could have been class valedictorian if he'd only applied himself; Duane had phenomenally high scores on all school aptitude tests. Duane attended a state university, largely because of Dave's urging. At State, Duane barely had a "C" average, his Ds and Fs compensated for by As in the courses he liked. He took five years to get his degree.

After graduating, Duane drifted from one job to another, usually winding up being dismissed for insubordination or undependability. He would dearly like to know what line of endeavor would be right for him, but he has no idea about what he wants to do, or even is able to do. He knows only one thing—that he doesn't want to enter the family business.

Dave is bitter about Duane's work and school history and feels betrayed and alienated because Duane has not lived up to—has apparently never even tried to live up to—his abundant promise. Dave has tried to talk to Duane about this on several occasions, but has always wound up these discussions by losing his temper and hurling accusations at Duane, who replies in kind before walking out on the scene.

Both men would like to see things different; neither knows how to go about changing the situation.

Why Children Are Thought to Fall Short

The world teems with individuals who haven't lived up to the expectations that others have held for them.

Reactions to this state of affairs vary. In the case of child and parent, both parties can be concerned or distressed about the apparent failure, sharing in the problem. Often the child is the victim of the parents' ambitions and will feel guilt, not so much about what he or she is doing as at disappointing the parents by letting them down. And sometimes the child is not concerned at all, either about personal achievment or about satisfying the parents, so that the problem rests entirely in the parents' laps.

Parents with adult children who appear to be misapplying, throwing away, or otherwise not using their talents effectively are particularly apt to indulge in self-blame. "We didn't do enough," "We didn't do the right things," "We were too easy," "We were too strict," the refrain may go, depending on the circumstances.

Whatever did or did not happen cannot be changed now, today, but it may help to realize that the Fall Short is one of the larger fictions of our time, often rooted in grave misunderstandings about the nature of individual abilities and their relationship to school and occupational performance.

Some of the misunderstanding originates with incomplete or distorted information. The uncritical partiality of parents is oftentimes validated by information that comes in from other quarters, especially teachers and counselors. Students take many tests in school and these tests are commonly used to form judgments about the child. Children who do well on tests of "intelligence" or "aptitude" are expected to perform well in school. The fact that the student has tested well and that high expectations are held for him or her is routinely communicated to the parents. Indeed, the schools use this information to move parents to motivate the child. If the child performs at a lower than predicted level, the parents are likely to be upset and get after the child. Nobody worries about "overachievers," the students who do better than might have been thought. Either that is fine or, alternatively, the performance is a fluke and things will even out over time.

There are several things wrong with this kind of thinking. The first thing wrong is that it puts intelligence at the pinnacle of the catalog of virtues. One of the peculiarities of American society is that it seems to value intelligence almost as extravagently as Aldous Huxley's Brave New World did. There is nothing the matter with intelligence, but crossed signals are found when people forget that:

1. There are several varieties of intelligence and having the kind of abilities that help in verbal-educational activities does not necessarily have anything profound to say about the individual's socioeconomic progress after school. One of the troubles with physicians these days may be that they are selected for medical school mainly on the basis of "intelligence." This makes them good students, but other kinds of intelligence have much to do with being a good practitioner. Overreliance on the intelligence test has harmed the general practice of medicine and certainly has eroded the high regard in which physicians used to be held.

2. Verbal-educational intelligence is only one small aspect of performance in any kind of activity, in or out of school. The relationship between verbal intelligence and school achievement, never very high, has been declining in the past few years; in the world of work a number of investigators report the relationship between intelligence and "success" to be slight, nil, or, in some instances, negative. This is not to say that intelligence is unimportant; it is simply no more important than a large collection of other factors involved in occupational success—work habits, interests, possession of special abilities, and personal attributes among them. Parents, teachers, and children err when they assume that verbal intelligence is the linchpin of success. It is not that, not even in forecasting school grades, the purpose for which verbal intelligence tests were originally developed.

3. Information about intelligence and other qualities comes from sources (teachers and counselors) who are not necessarily qualified to evaluate and convey this sort of information. Teachers will have had brief training in the principles of testmaking, but ordinarily will not have a close understanding of the topic; counselors will have had a bit more training, but not enough to deal with or explain this complex subject comfortably.

What teachers or counselors have to say about the abilities of students may be quite inaccurate, based on misunderstandings or misinterpretations, or, worse, they may misrepresent the student. Teachers sometimes advance evaluations of students for their presumed effect on parents, issuing inflated communiques about abilities or potentialities in the hope that this well-meant distortion will induce the parent to motivate the student to work harder and better. "With a bit more effort, Janey could be getting all 'A's." The point of all this is that estimates of potential are almost certain to be incomplete, one-sided, and possibly exaggerated. Even when they are fair, complete, and accurate portrayals, they will have only a modest relationship to later performance. The Fall Short is often the victim of misleading labeling.

4. The predictive accuracy of tests has always been measured by studying groups. Applying information derived from such group analysis to individual cases is a method suffering serious logical flaws.

There are other problems beyond incomplete, distorted, or mischievously overblown estimates of talent. Adult children do not live up to their potentialities for a variety of reasons, some of which have been set forth in discussing the reasons for the Unemptied Nest phenomenon. Beyond that, there is the problem of deciding what represents performance consistent with potential. What indeed is "success?"

Apart from the fallibility of information about children and their performances, other broader social trends also enter into the picture. One of them has been what amounts to a partial rejection, by children, of parental values. Preoccupation with security and material well-being in the parental generation has, in many instances, been supplanted by the decision to "do right" rather than to "do well." Parents want (and want their children) to live well; the children may want to live right according to their lights. Living right may involve doing things that strain the powers of the parents to understand and

accept—working for causes or issues, living according to eco-
logical precepts, and so on. Parents who have worked hard
and sacrificed to enjoy their comfort and security are inclined
to believe that what has been good enough for them ought to
be good enough for their offspring, rejecting the argument
that the gravest threat to our materialistic, consumption-ori-
ented society is unrestrained materialism and consumerism.
Many young adults do understand this, and in accepting it are
led to reject some of the values and habits of their progenitors.

Somewhat related to this point is the curious view that
many parents—especially male parents—take of themselves.
They believe that each generation ought to surpass in its
accomplishments those of the preceding generation. Ever on-
ward, ever upward. They disregard, if they were ever aware
of the simple statistical fact, that in half of cases the children
will have less of any ability that the parents display. Dave, in
our example, reflects this—out of a working-class background, he moved up by dint of hard work (and the GI Bill.)

Dave wants and expects Duane to surpass his own considerable attainments. After all, Duane has had more advantages and possesses better abilities ("intelligence") than he
had. Why shouldn't Duane turn out to be someone really significant—a university president, a judge, a surgeon—some-
body who would make a difference? A strange kind of push-
pull motivational technique is at work in cases such as this,
one in which the parent simultaneously urges the child to new
heights of effort and attainment, while downgrading or making light of the parent's own accomplishments. Once you've
accomplished something, the parents who take this tack seem
to be saying, it's easy and no longer especially important.

The children know better. They have seen how hard the
Daves of the world work, how much time and energy they
devote to their occupation, its demands and their sacrifices.
They see that the Daves have little time for fun, for recreation.
They are aware of the overriding commitment to the occupa-

tion. Some develop serious doubts about whether they could or should make those kinds of sacrifices. In addition they have understandable doubts about their ability to match what the Daves have done, and they see no need to, or sense in, competing with their fathers. So they withdraw, realizing that bettering the old man's track record may demand more of them than they want to put out, so they settle for a less stressful, less demanding course of action.

An important, if fallible, article of faith has it that there is a square hole for every square peg and that it is somehow wrong for the individual not to be placed precisely in a situation in which he or she will be performing at the zenith of competence. Only now are we beginning to put aside this spectacularly wrong and hideously destructive idea—yet another unhappy consequence of our technological society— that there is one best direction for any individual to head in life. This belief denies that the individual is multipotentialed and flexible, and almost certainly can perform capably in a wide range of roles. Caliber of performance is determined not only by factors inhering in the individual, but by the larger economic and social context and the particular work environment to which the individual is exposed. Work is carried out in a social milieu that can make it enjoyable and rewarding, even if it does not call out a high level of training, great skill, or life and death responsibility.

Social status is partly defined by work. It remains a dominant consideration for the older generation. For them, occupational prestige ties most closely to economic returns. A good job carries responsibility and demands effort to be sure, but most important, it pays off.

When children cut themselves off from this flow of economic goods, questions begin to pop up. Relatives or friends become curious and (without intending it) patronizingly sympathetic when Janey, with all that promise, gets along doing something anybody at all can do. And it never helps when the smug word comes out that your klutzy nephew finished dental school and is earning God knows how much per annum.

To recap, the first thing to consider when faced with a Fall Short is the possibility that the child is not falling short at all. You may be operating under the burden of inappropriate, overstated, or distorted expectations. After all, that the child may not be a latter-day Einstein does not make him or her any less worthy of or entitled to your love and support.

Similarly, that the child is extremely bright does not guarantee anything. Performance in school, as in the world, requires more than verbal intelligence alone. It is not only what you know and whom you know, but where, how, and why you use what you know that adds up to what you are. Potential is merely that—the capacity to perform in a given way if the conditions are right.

I once spent two summers building a home in the mountains. I had people come in at various times to help. One of my helpers was and is a "genius." He understands the principles of physics perfectly (he has a degree with highest honors in the field), but could not be taught how to use a spade with any skill or proficiency at all. He wanted to learn and help. But it was beyond his physical capabilities. Knowing the law of the lever and knowing how to use a lever are simply different acts that require different talents.

The idea that a child is failing, then, may result from unrealistic expectations on the parts of the parents. Each generation has expected the succeeding one to match or surpass its own accomplishments. Given that children, in half of all instances, will not be as talented as their parents, and that the competition for rungs at the top of the ladder has intensified, the need for an ever-upward spiral of accomplishment becomes a clear, though obviously impossible, ideal. The frontier has vanished; we are in an era when we must confront our real limits.

Even if it were possible, an increasing number of young persons today do not seem willing to expend the effort, time, and sacrifice needed to achieve the ideal of success held by their parents. A friend recounted this story to me:

> Responding to the intense, unrelenting pressure from his parents, a young man completed medical school. He did this to satisfy his parents, but he had never had and still does not have a wish to practice medicine. At the time, the friend told me that he was in training to become a medical technician, work that appealed to him and would enable him to live the kind of life he wants. He has come to terms with himself, but the parents cannot comprehend what has led to this "crazy" decision. They are upset with his plans and feel that their sacrifices are to no avail and unappreciated. They have even thought seriously of suing their son to recover the costs of his education.

Putting Ambition in Perspective

This section is about the ambitions and expectations that parents have for their children or that children have for themselves. We are of course fallible in our expectations, and when they are miscalculated, they are much more likely to err on the high side. Hopes are always extravagant, the more so because they have no limits.

Being disappointed because a child has not become all you wanted, or that he or she might have wished, paves a freeway to despair. "The saddest words of tongue or pen..." Dwelling on your children's misses, near or not so near, on their failures, on their misfires, can all too readily become a way of life. It is quite possible—and considerably more pleasant and satisfying—to try to focus on the positive accomplishments of your offspring.

This seemingly blithe suggestion is of course more easily offered than accepted. With effort, it is quite possible to program yourself primarily to look for, share in, and value the successful, the affirmative things that your children do or become. Congratulations or support can spring to tongue as readily as criticism or condemnation, and always have more agreeable consequences. For parents with unrealistically high goals for their children, this perhaps somewhat Panglossian prescription may be swallowed only with difficulty, especially when so much importance is attached to competition and success. Even if it does go down, nothing save personal sweetness may come of it. But the very effort to be largely positive, largely affirmative in tone may help clear out some of your externally defined, culturally determined ideas of success, thus ridding you of any undue anxiety and concern about what your children are making of themselves. You may become much more ready to recognize their viewpoints—and their rights and responsibilities—as adults. And you may also begin to understand that your ambitions for your children—founded on an understandable and laudable concern for their well-being—may well reflect your own camouflaged desire to relive your life and rectify your own failures through their successes. In that framework, when they don't manage to attain the goals you project for them, your own burden of failure is increased. You don't need that. Recognizing the valid accomplishments and respecting the rights and responsibilities of your children will greatly lighten your load.

Getting Help

When parent and child accept the view that accomplishment has fallen short of potential, and when the causes and remedies are not self-evident, the procedures for locating outside help parallel those suggested for the Unemptied Nest. In fact, the Fall Short represents a special case of that problem. However, it is useful to begin by getting a thorough, competent, and unbiased inventory of the child's capabilities, providing there is agreement on your and the child's part regarding the need for it. This cataloging of aptitudes, skills, interests, and other attributes can generally be carried out through a college or university counseling center, many of which offer just such services to the public, as well as the university community, for a nominal fee. Psychologists in private practice as vocational or educational counselors provide similar assessments, but should always be checked out beforehand to establish their qualifications and fees.

Getting good information about your child may represent something of a difficulty because, ethically, personal data belong to the individual directly involved, that is, the child, not the parent. If the child agrees to share these data—or if you become involved in a joint counseling arrangement—this hurdle can be bypassed, but it will still pay to remember that it is the right of the child to have personal information kept in confidence.

With a somewhat more complete, honest, and independent assessment of the child's abilities, entry into a program of career planning would be the next step. Bolles' approach, already described, is recommended for this purpose.

When the problem resides largely in the minds of the parents, and causes substantial unhappiness and discord, some sessions of individual or group counseling in an appropriate setting may help bring about greater understanding, acceptance, and some degree of emancipation from the harsh values the parental culture imposes.

Finally, keep in mind that the best anyone can do is to broaden the information base that you and the child possess.

How talent is to be used—and what is an appropriate level at which to employ it—remains a decision that the child, whether alone or with help, must always make personally.

CHAPTER 8

MEDDLESOME GRANDPARENTS

Being a grandparent is the best revenge.

Introduction

Middle-aged parents sometimes find themselves uncomfortably caught in the middle of a struggle between their own parents and their adult children—a shared problem straddling three generations.

Any and all of the kinds of difficulties young people are heir to can and do provide grist for this sort of dilemma. Only the decline of the nuclear family and the geographical separation of its members keep it from being more prevalent and troublesome than it already is.

The Stone family has three Tims—Tim Sr., the grandfather, his only son, Tim Jr., and the grandson, Tim III, who is twenty-five. GrandfatherStone remains a vigorous, opinionated man at seventy-eight. When his wife died eleven years ago, he moved to be closer to the only family he had left—his son, his daughter-in-law, and the grandchildren. He spends a fair amount of time with them, dropping by several times a week to visit, often staying on for meals and to watch TV. He has always been especially interested in Tim III, who is the only grandson and his namesake.

115

Tim III has never shown much interest in the kinds of leisure activities the rest of the family enjoys—sports, and outdoor activities especially. From childhood he was bookish, spending his free hours reading. He became interested in drawing, was encouraged to develop his talent by his teachers, and went on to major in art in college. He works as a design and layout artist for a large advertising firm. Tim III has never ceased to puzzle and trouble the old man, who cannot understand the direction of his interests and his work. The grandfather fears that the grandson is homosexual and that the Stone line will die out with him. He blames Tim Jr. for this imaginary state of affairs and continually urges him to do something about it. Whenever he sees Tim III (who no longer lives at home), he constantly grills the grandson with such questions as "Tim, about time you were getting married, isn't it? Got any plans?"

Tim III, who is fond of the old man and not homosexual, puts off these questions with joking, noncommittal answers that only fuel the old man's apprehensions. Tim Jr. began experiencing such feelings of anger and annoyance at his father's continual harping on the subject of Young Tim that he began to avoid him, sometimes to the point of calling ahead to see whether the old man was there. If so, he would either stay at the office or find refuge in a nearby bar until the coast was clear. This put the brunt of the grief on the wife, Moira, who wound up resenting both her husband and her father-in-law.

Matters finally reached the point that Tim Jr. sought me out to get help with what was proving to be a strifetorn mess.

In my experience, gratuitous advice and critical second-guessing about the method and results of the upbringing of grandchildren all too often produces its own measure of intergenerational tension in families. It may batten upon and aggravate an existing concern of the parents so that the problem, whatever it is, is blown far out of proportion to its actual severity. It also creates conflict between grandparent and parent, conflict that is especially difficult to resolve constructively and amicably because of generational differences and the disposition of some elders to grow "set in their ways." Notwithstanding that the process of aging is accompanied by a tendency to become more conservative on social and other issues, there is no reason to believe that the "old-old" are incapable of receiving and acting reflectively and flexibly on information properly presented.

In a sense the two younger Stones brought on the problem because they failed to address Tim Sr.'s concerns directly. Though they love and respect him, they tend to treat him with the tolerant, amused indulgence that our society seems to reserve for the very young, the not so bright, and the old. One of the worst things about being old is no longer being taken seriously.

After a few interviews with Tim Jr., the facts sketched above emerged. Moreover, it also became evident that Tim Sr. was still intellectually and emotionally intact. I advised Tim Jr. to talk first with Tim III, and then to discuss the matter directly and openly with the grandfather. I cautioned them that the old man's attitudes about homosexuality were probably so deeply rooted and antipathetic that he would likely deny vehemently that that issue had anything to do with the matter. Here I badly underestimated the old gentleman, who openly aired his concerns.

The meeting went extremely well, mainly because Tim III spoke forthrightly and affectionately to his grandfather, acknowledging that perhaps he was not all that his grandfather might have desired, but that sometimes he wished that the old man would be more understanding and tolerant of him, too. This criticism, gently given, came with reassurances about Tim III's heterosexuality and the reminder that Tim III had the right to make his own life decisions. The message got through to Tim Sr. and matters improved significantly at once.

Not all problems with grandparents are resolved quite as smoothly as the one involving the three Tims. Because it turned out that the problem existed only in Tim Sr.'s imagination, it was therefore able to be disposed of readily by direct discussion. Some of his underlying fears—for instance, perpetuation of the family name, a matter or real concern for the old man—persist, but with the context greatly changed, they no longer seriously upset the others concerned.

Dealing Constructively with Grandparental Conflict

Opening up the lines of communication—the first goal in any intergenerational conflict—sometimes may not be possible. When there has been physical or psychological deterioration the needs and concerns of the oldster may become obsessive, overriding not only respect for the rights of others, but also the importance of basing actions on evidence, the need for justice, and the hope for a sense of fair play in relationships between individuals. When the capacity to honor these values is absent, is seriously diminished, or perhaps never existed, the middle-aged parent is faced with a difficult situation.

Happily, most older people do not manifest symptoms of a seriously disabling deterioration. Though our elders are likely to show some loss of sensory sharpness—visual problems, reduced acuity of hearing, a dulling of taste and smell—these testaments to the process of aging are not crippling, but essentially only disquieting. However, in some instances aging has its psychological correlates, too. One common companion to old age is depression which, as Erikson notes, is likely to result when the individual in the last of the "eight ages" fails to integrate the cumulative experience of the past. This failure to come to terms with the realities of the elder's life all too often brings a concomitant depression or despair.

Some of the physical changes during aging do produce psychological effects. Alterations in the circulatory system that bring on sclerotic conditions can profoundly affect the level or span of attention and may produce a consistent irascibility or petulance. Memory may be impaired so that the conversations of the individual often become repetitive or fragmentary and hard to follow.

Depression in either the old or young may inspire aggravated self-concern, fear, and withdrawal, interfering with the ability to communicate openly and constructively. And older persons experiencing these transformations in personality and loss of ability to communicate almost always become less flexible, less able to accommodate to novelty or change. There is little that can be done to restore their adaptive capacity; you, their middle-aged child, will simply have to find the requisite personal resources of understanding and tolerance to accept these irreversible developments. The only other alternative, breaking off contact, sometimes seems inviting, but this tactic would certainly not be understood, would not address the central problem, and would have destructive, demoralizing consequences for you and your parent. When your parent is part of a problem involving your own children, and seems unlikely to be able to deal with it constructively, when his or her attitudes have pushed you into ever greater difficulty, the initiatives for change must come from you. Adjustments or modifications occur only when they are possible, and outside help, which can indeed provide you a different perspective and help you to develop different strategies for dealing with a problem, is often especially beneficial.

With a real problem, that is, one in which the grandparent is upset and causing further distress about the unacceptable behavior of grandchildren—a situation in which all three generations are caught in the same dilemma—other strategies are needed.

This rather more complicated state of affairs requires, as do most other problems in our lives, open communication and careful, dispassionate analysis. The principles involved

here are identical with those applied to other problems encountered elsewhere—first, define the issue; second, locate it
(in the three generation problem, there are seven possible
loci); and third, work out a course of action based on the possible solutions and their consequences, taking into account
the rights and responsibilities of all those involved. The parent—here unluckily occupying the middle—will probably
need to launch the process.

It sometimes happens that grandchildren find it easier to
discuss or open up about their problems with grandparents.
In those circumstances the grandparent may have the awkward task of informing the parent of a difficulty and then
helping both child and parent deal with it. More often, however, the grandparent will either disapprove of the actions of
a grandchild and the way that the parent is attending to them,
or the child will resent the intervention of the grandparent. In
general, the grandparental generation is less likely to tolerate
or condone departures from older ideals of sexual morality,
although attitudes and responses do vary widely, depending
on the individual concerned.

Getting Help

One rarely hears of a very old person consulting a psychologist or psychiatrist. This is not because older people live
problem-free lives—any time of life has its own complement
of troubles and old age has rather more than most. However,
psychotherapy is the province of the young and the grandparental generation gets along with its problems as best it can.
This aversion to psychotherapy may stem in part from the
stigma older people attach to it. But it also grows out of other
things—costs, the settled conviction that it does no good, or
the belief that it is an admission of weakness.

Psychotherapy aims to help the individual to function
better in relation to other individuals or institutions—school

work, marriage, family—and most curiously seems to be regarded as irrelevant for older people. The idea of irrelevance may perhaps stem from the notion underlying the adage about being unable to teach old dogs new tricks, but that particular bit of folk wisdom happens to be false. Older individuals experience, and most of them adapt to, the cruelest kinds of losses—decline in physical vigor, the deaths of friends and loved ones—so that invoking psychological aid at the time the crisis is at its most severe would seem to promise considerable help in surmounting it.

Other potential helping sources that may be particularly appropriate and effective for older individuals include religious figures (priests, ministers, rabbis, and so on), physicians, support groups, relatives, trusted friends, as well any of the ancillary resources outlined in Chapter 20. If an individual resists seeking assistance, either because of a settled conviction that he or she is right, or that seeking help is a sign of weakness or personal failure, or if there has been deterioration to the extent that outside assistance would be pointless, then the responsibility for solving the problem shifts to the others involved. They must somehow learn to live with the trouble the oldster represents.

Chapter 9

INJURY AND ILLNESS

When sorrows come, they come not single spies, but in battalions.

Introduction

Injury or illness can keep a child dependent for a lifetime; it can also abruptly transform an independent into a dependent child—one with overwhelming problems and needs. Moreover, adult children who suddenly become disabled will often have their own dependents who then become complicating elements in what is already a complex and difficult situation.

The list of conditions that can be responsible for serious disability is long and growing. For every disease that yields to scientific or medical advances, another baffling one seems to spring up to replace it. More hazardous conditions of life—the automobile to take one instance—make certain kinds of disabling injuries much more common, whereas medical advances help prolong the lives of persons who are severely impaired. Moreover, the growing toxicity of the environment is responsible for increasing the incidence of cancer, of neurological and associated psychological disorders, and of diseases associated with compromise of the immune system.

In some instances, the child never quite stops being a dependent:

Bobby was a problem from the moment he was born. His parents couldn't get him on a schedule; he always seemed restless and cried incessantly. He had trouble with school right from the start, not doing well, not liking it, having both academic and behavioral problems. He began exhibiting strange and upsetting behavior in junior high school and was diagnosed as schizophrenic when in his late teens. Now 27, he lives at home. He has been hospitalized a number of times for varying periods, has tried unsuccessfully to be on his own, but has been unable to make it in group care situations. At best he is reclusive and moody; he takes offense quickly, becomes argumentative and resentful at the slightest provocation. He sometimes experiences delusions or hallucinations, and he be comes agitated for no apparent reason. He needs supervision to keep himself groomed and clean. He is on a heavy regimen of medications that, when he takes them, keep him quiet, but reduce him to a state of near stupor.

In other instances, the disability happens with overwhelming suddenness:

Ann and Wes have three kids. The older two, a son and a daughter, are on their own, married, and getting along fine; Kenny, the youngest, now 23, was just getting started two years ago. He was working as a carpenter, liked it, enjoyed being out on his own. Then, one August evening, Kenny, his friend Paul, and their girlfriends went to the county fair in Paul's pickup truck, Kenny and his date riding in the back.

They attended the fair, had a good time, drank a few beers, took in the Midway, and then piled in the truck to come home. On the way out of the fairgrounds Paul had to brake suddenly to avoid hitting another car that cut in ahead of him. He was only doing about 20 miles per hour, but the sudden deceleration caught Kenny by surprise. It threw him sideways—he was sitting on the wheel well—and propelled him into the rear of the cab. The impact broke his neck. He has been a quadriplegic from that moment. He has lived at home since he got out of the hospital and has tried to become independent, but it has been a hard struggle for him. It has been hard for Ann and Wes, too. Not only has care of Kenny been physically and psychologically demanding, but it has been costly as well. Just to make their home wheelchair-accessible cost them over $10,000.

Disability in Perspective

Disability in an adult child is likely to be a problem that child and parent will share, at least to some extent. Whether the disability is recent or of long standing, parents are often inclined to and can usually find a way of blaming themselves for it. This parental guilt—or shame in the cases of disabilities that people don't like to talk about—is often accompanied by equally serious and complicating emotional upsets in the disabled offspring; profound depression, anger, anxiety.

I cannot possibly cover all of the various conditions that can and do cause disabilities in young adults.

- There are literally hundreds of them and they arise from any of a myriad of genetic, psychogenic, or sociogenic causes, as well as disease or injury
- They may range in severity from quite intractable to quite treatable
- They can differ enormously in the extent to which they impair the individual
- They can represent such a monumental problem or challenge that they all but immobilize the parents
- They can offer the opportunity for significant growth, accomplishment, and satisfaction under what would seem like the most unlikely and trying of circumstances

Strategies for Dealing with a Disabled Child

Coping with a disabled adult child entails devising and adopting a strategy that addresses the needs of both parent and child. What specific steps you, the middle-aged parent, will take in response to a disabled child will vary, depending on the nature of the disability and the individuals involved. However, you will have to face up to and act on a number of tough questions. Here are some of the more obvious ones:

1. Do you want to get involved? To what extent?

2. Has your child's problem been evaluated medically? If so, what is the medical status? Are you satisfied with the evaluation? Are insurance companies or Workers' Compensation involved? What are the medical rights and entitlements in this instance?

3. Have the financial aspects and alternatives of the problem been explored? Is there eligibility for or entitlement to assistance from the state, SSI, insurance carriers, Workers' Compensation, Unemployment?

4. Have the legal aspects of the situation been explored, especially in the case of work-related injury or illness?

5. Is rehabilitation or retraining feasible? Available? Is the child motivated to undertake it? In what ways can you help to motivate him or her?

6. Help sources for the care and rehabilitation of the child are available if looked for diligently. What sources does your community have? Physical or occupational therapy? Have they been tapped? Transportation? Home care or nursing?

7. Have you sought help and support for yourself?

Getting the answers to each of these questions will take time, persistence, and patience in dealing with the many individuals and agencies that are likely to be involved. For the parents of disabled children, acting on the first and last of these questions is imperative because they define what your role is likely to be and whether or not you can sustain it. The next sections of this chapter outline approaches to answering these two questions.

Do You Want to Get Involved?

This question implies that you have some options, which may not be entirely true if the problem is a long-standing one, as in the case of Bobby. It also assumes that your help has been requested, and this might not be the case. The disabled child may have the resources to go it alone without parental help. If so, fine! When your help has not been requested and is not sought, the wise parent will avoid getting involved.

When help is requested or the need for it is determined to exist, you will next have to decide whether you are willing to pitch in. If you cannot, say so and give your reasons, whatever they may be—time, distance, lack of money or resources, conflicting obligations, and physical or health limitations.

If you can help, you will next have to determine whether you are capable of carrying through with what is being asked. However, it is often difficult to know this in advance and people facing these situations tend to assume considerably more responsibility than they can readily fulfill. Moreover, they often fail to use available resources, such as attendant care. In short, you must be brutally realistic about just how far your material, physical, and psychological resources will stretch. Caring for another person can be immensely rewarding; it can also be demeaning, confining, frustrating, physically demanding, and enormously stressful.

You know yourself, your limits, and the other obligations you are carrying. If you decide that there are limits to what you can or are willing to do, it is essential to state them, and then to try to create a situation in which both you and your child's needs are well-attended to, even if it proves necessary to call in outside resources. The steps traced in Figure 2 will

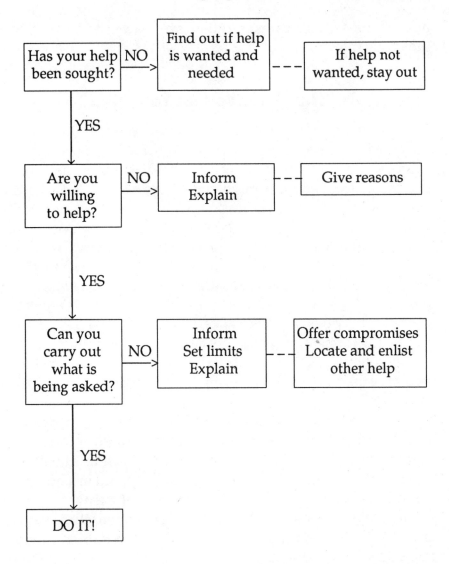

Fig. 2. Steps in deciding whether or not to help

help you decide whether and to what extent you will be able to help.

Have You Sought Help and Support for Yourself?

Depending on the nature and extent of your involvement with a disabled child, you yourself may need or might benefit from any of a variety of outside helping sources. Those that provide direct assistance with physical care, retraining, rehabilitation, and material support are listed in Chapter 20. In addition, and perhaps more important, you may require aid in dealing with the feelings that even a limited amount of responsibility for the care of a disabled person provokes. This sort of psychological buoying up can be supplied by conventional help sources—friends, clergymen, counselors, relatives —but their efforts can be substantially abetted by support groups that bring together individuals caring for those with specific disabilities. In communities of any size at all, you are likely to find support groups of care providers for persons with AIDS, anorexia and bulimia, autism, blindness, cancer, cardiac or coronary problems, cystic fibrosis, deafness, epilepsy or seizure disorders, head trauma, learning disabilities, multiple sclerosis, ostomy, Parkinson's disease, schizophrenia and other psychiatric disorders, spinal cord injury, and stroke, as well as many other specific chronic diseases or disabilities.

In addition, your community will, in all likelihood, have agencies that exist primarily to promote the independence of the disabled. Independent Living Skills Programs and Centers, where people with disabilities are helped to become competent in personal, social, and household management, are becoming increasingly common, and other organizations, such as Goodwill, are devoted to the welfare of disabled individuals and are a fixture in most places. Beyond providing valuable services directly, these groups also offer various programs designed to assist nondisabled persons who are responsible for or involved in the ongoing care of the disabled.

Independence for Disabled Children

More than 200 Centers for Independent Living have now sprung up all over the United States. These Centers have made us aware of an extremely important truth—that most people with disabilities can manage quite competently on their own despite expectations to the contrary.

It often happens that when this potential for living independently is not realized, the parents of the disabled person are the key obstacle. Out of understandable feelings of attachment, responsibility, or fear of what might happen in their absence, they hold the child back, standing in the way of him or her becoming a fully independent being with an autonomous life.

Letting go of a child is difficult under any circumstances; when that child is disabled, the decision can become even more troubling. Yet, it is inevitable that the separation will occur at some point. You can be most helpful as a parent by encouraging and aiding your adult child toward an independence of body and spirit—an independence that accepts no false limits or arbitrary constraints.

CHAPTER 10

STEPPARENTS AND STEPCHILDREN

I didn't expect it to turn out to be like the Brady Bunch—but this?—this is ridiculous!

Introduction

People marry, have children, and these days, quite often divorce.

Divorced people remarry and when they do, the children of the earlier marriage inevitably become a part of the new arrangement. They may also become a particularly rich and troublesome source of problems. Any category of problem that bedevils other children may also afflict stepchildren. They can also be the focus of tension and stress in the family— tension and stress that arise from their special status as step-children. This chapter deals with some of the difficulties that crop up between stepparents and stepchildren. For obvious reasons, it does not dwell on the fact—one deserving mention here—that stepparents and stepchildren more often than not find one another sources of love and delight.

Since this book concerns itself with middle-aged parents and their grown children, it does not address the difficult task of rearing minor stepchildren, surely one of the more complex

chores that any couple can assume. When stepchildren are
concerned, the ordinary rights and responsibilities of parents
become more complicated, both by the existence of an absent
parent or parents who have legal and familial ties to the children, and by the attitudes of the children toward the new
arrangement. And similarly, when divorced parents with
grown children remarry, knotty problems with the grownup
stepchildren can be one of the unexpected dividends.

Marian had four children during her initial marriage. Her
first husband abandoned her when the kids were still quite
young. She remarried and Tom, the second husband, and she
could not agree on how the children, especially the next to the
youngest, a boy, were to be disciplined. Matters came to a
head when Tom sold the boy's car—a car that the boy had
bought and supported out of money that he earned—after the
boy, then 17, was involved in a minor traffic accident. Marian
walked out at that point, taking the son and the youngest
daughter with her. A divorce ensued and three years later
Marian married Jerry, who had been divorced years before
and had two grown daughters of his own. Jerry's daughters
intensely dislike and refuse to have anything at all to do with
Marian. To them it's as if she doesn't even exist, and Marian is
deeply wounded by their attitude. Marian's children pose a
problem for Jerry, too, because the second child, a daughter
with two young children of her own, has had her marriage
fail. After that divorce she came down with a serious chronic
illness that has kept her from working. She has become dependent on Marian for financial help and for child care when
she is not able to look after her kids. Jerry didn't bargain for
two rambunctious stepgrandsons. He resents the loss of freedom and privacy, and begrudges the money Marian "lends"
her daughter even though it comes from her earnings as partner in a very successful real estate firm. Though counseling
has helped Marian and Jerry to bring out and discuss their
feelings openly, there is still considerable unhappiness and
strain associated with the other's children.

The Authority Problem

When difficulties exist between stepchildren and step-parents, the nub of the problem is likely to be found in disagreements about what amounts to proper stepfilial responsibility or legitimate stepparental authority.

"So long as you're in my house you'll do as I say."

"You're not my mother. You have no right to tell me how to act."

When the child is in the home, stepparents are likely to have a parental role thrust on them, assuming at least some of the responsibility for nurturing and guiding the child. The stepchild, troubled, perhaps puzzled by the splitup of its natural parents, may somehow feel at fault, confused by divided loyalties, unsure about its place or role. The stepparent may be blamed unfairly for the failure of the marriage and whatever plight the absent parent is in. All of these convoluted difficulties make it easy for problems to surface—even if the relationship between child and natural parent is solid and free of strain. And, where stepchildren are involved, it is particularly important to get down to the core problem.

The analytic steps and procedures presented in Chapter 4 are especially relevant here.

Stepchild–Stepparent Relationships

The relationship between stepchild and stepparent can be thought of as falling in to one of four categories, depending on the attitudes stepchild and stepparent bear toward one another.

Stepparent attitude toward stepchild	Stepchild attitude toward stepparent	
	Accepting	Rejecting
Accepting	1	2
Rejecting	3	4

If the stepparent's and stepchild's attitudes toward one another are essentially accepting—category 1 in the grid sketched above—then there is no special problem, apart from the usual ones having to do with middle-aged parents and their natural grown children.

Each of the other combinations does, however, represent a distinct kind of quandary that calls for its own approach, but nonetheless always relies heavily on the natural parent as the mediator.

Category 2, in which the stepparent's attitude is accepting, but the stepchild's is rejecting, permits alternative strategies. On the one hand the attitude can simply be accepted for what it is and accommodated by arranging contacts or activities accordingly. This is an awkward, uncomfortable situation, but it may represent the best compromise when feelings are deep and bitter. It carries the risk of straining relationships between the stepparent and the natural parent or of distancing parent and child, and cannot be regarded as a wholly satisfactory alternative.

A second approach is one that strives to bring the stepchild and stepparent together. This entails trying to discover the source or cause of the child's feelings and taking steps to resolve them. Since the feelings are likely to be complex, incompletely understood, and possibly arise out of causes that are unknown or repressed, this may be difficult to achieve and long in coming.

After a short illness Sarah's father died when she was 19 and a sophomore in college. Her mother, Lillian, remarried a year later. The new stepfather, a childless widower, was delighted at the prospect of having a family. Sarah, who had been extremely close to her father, was furious at what she regarded as her mother's betrayal of her father and treated the stepfather with resentment and contempt that she made no effort to conceal. She was having so much trouble with her feelings that they began to interfere with her academic performance and she came to me for help. Over the course of a year she grew to understand and resolved much of the anger she felt toward her mother. In time, she gradually accepted the stepfather, becoming in a real sense, the daughter that the stepfather had hoped to have.

The variation on the stepchild–stepparent theme in which the stepparent rejects the child—category 3 in the table—presents alternatives similar to those that apply to the preceding case. You can, of course, arrange your life to skirt the feelings, an evasive step that fails to address the underlying problem even while it promotes discord between husband and wife. Alternatively, you can try to understand the reasons for the rejection, and then work at developing strategies for dealing with or overcoming them directly. Here the suggestions about defining and understanding problems that appear in Chapter 4 will be useful to you.

Feelings of rejection in a stepchild or stepparent are often an amalgam of many different elements. The child may feel guilt or responsibility for the breakup of the natural parents' marriage; anger at the parent who remarries for having let down the other parent; grief for the loss of the other parent; resentment at the stepparent for having seduced the parent. Elements of hurt, anxiety, and even cupidity may enter in.

> Irene has two sons, Brt and Earl. Her husband died when the boys were in their thirties. After being alone for five years she married Rob who, everyone agrees, is a "great guy." Everyone except Burt, that is. Burt, even though he is very well off, loathes Rob because he sees Rob as getting "his" inheritance.

From the stepparent's side, the child may represent an unwanted or unanticipated obligation, or even an irksome reminder of other times and connections. Jealousy often enters in.

On either side, there may be a real dislike of the other person. Certainly the sense of connectedness, of being "related" is not present, at least at the outset, and much of the time it never develops. One tends to hear references to "his kids" or "her kids" rather than to "my stepkids."

It frequently happens that the individual harboring the negative feelings—child or stepparent—seems intransigent when it comes to doing something about them. Under that circumstance the best one can do is to open up lines of communication in the least provocative or threatening fashion possible and then to work toward a suitable compromise. When honest respect or liking is impossible, simple civility may be the only option. When the stepchild is the intransigent, the absent parent, siblings, or other relatives may help to illuminate the rights and responsibilities of all those involved. There are, so far as I know, no support groups for adult stepchildren, but such groups do exist for both adolescents and stepparents.

For the stepparent, overcoming the rejection of the stepchild may represent an even greater stumbling block because middle-aged people, unlike younger folks, are little given to opening up their feelings to the possiblity of change, and thus are more likely to believe that right is on their side.

In the worst-possible-case scenario, when a stepparent and a stepchild are mutually antagonistic—category 4—the tendency probably is to let matters alone. This approach, though it dodges confrontation and appears to avoid making matters worse (not that they can't get worse on their own), invites continuing friction and dissension between parent and stepparent. Time is not always the great healer. In this unhappy situation, a procedure in which each of the parties works independently to define the problem and to examine the rights and responsibilities of the individuals involved, followed by a joint discussion moderated by a neutral party who is respected, trusted by, and acceptable to everyone, might possibly work. This moderator might best be a clergyman, a relative, a mutual friend, teacher, or counselor.

Prenuptial Agreements

One tactic that is often successful in warding off serious personality clashes between stepparents and stepchildren is to arrive at an understanding before the marriage takes place. Children would know of the plan to marry and be asked to identify and help work out those aspects of the marriage that affect them. Depending on the circumstances, such an agreement might cover property settlements, educational arrangements, domiciling and visitation (where and with whom to spend holidays is often a big issue for stepchildren and stepparents), financial and other aspects of support, and so on. During this process it should be made clear that the decision to marry is not on the table. The right of the older couple to marry, or to live together if that is the case, is theirs alone to exercise. But having the children know of the plan, having them know of the reasons for it and the feelings behind it, having them aware that it has been seriously thought through, and making clear to them that they played a part in the process—all of these things do help to define, clarify, and formalize the various relationships involved, thus anticipating and blunting some potentially stressful problems.

Stepchild vs Stepchild

One of the more melancholy aspects of our heritage is the consistent portrayal, in myth or fairy tale, of the stepparent or stepsibling as wicked, cruel, greedy, vindictive. This destructive stereotype probably predisposes stepchildren from two marriages to dislike one another. Disagreements between stepchildren, usually accompanied by each believing that the other (natural) children are being accorded preferential treatment, are quite commonplace.

It is probably wrong to expect parents—young or old—to be perfectly even-handed in their treatment of natural and stepchildren; even natural siblings generally believe they are not treated equally in the family. Among stepchildren, not only are the relationships different, but after all, blood is thicker than water. However, it is highly desirable to avoid strife and bitterness between sets of stepchildren, and the parents ought always to work consciously at being fair and equitable in their treatment of the children. Though matters of discipline, the bane of families with younger, at-home step-kids, are not so likely to trouble older parents, there will be the usual pleas for family help and support. When this happens the matters of how, in what way, and how much to assist, of the source and limits of aid, and so on must be carefully reckoned and made known. Fairness, consistency, and honesty in dealing with children (natural or step-) will help to avoid conflict. Children are not naturally disposed to dislike one another, but stepparents concentrating on their own fresh beginnings can fail to pay proper attention to their concerns, and turn a situation needlessly sour.

Parents should also know and clearly communicate whatever it is they expect from their own children in the way of behavior. Common courtesy and respect for the rights of others is certainly the minimum to which one might reasonably aspire.

Getting Help

When there are personality conflicts between adult parents and grown stepchildren, the natural parent may feel especially threatened. If informal sources (friends, relatives) are unavailable or cannot help, one should look for (if the spouse agrees to participate) a qualified (licensed) family counselor. If the marital partner is not willing to participate, then the concerned parent should either look for an individual counselor or join a men's or women's support group for those working through situations similar to your own. Hearing how others have been affected by such problems, seeing how they may have gone about solving their difficulties, learning the blunders and pitfalls to avoid—all of these can provide a powerful learning experience that will enable you to cope successfully with this—or any other—class of problem you may confront.

In addition to doing whatever can be done to solve or reduce the severity of the problem directly, conflict involving stepchildren is especially likely to provoke stress, so that the stress-managing or stress-reducing procedures presented in Chapter 3 are good to know about and to put into practice.

CHAPTER 11

LEGAL, FISCAL, AND OTHER PLIGHTS

*I do not love him because he is good,
but because he is my little child.*

Introduction

Children, being human, get into scrapes. Today it seems easier than ever for adult children to stumble into difficulty.

In the situations described below, the children got themselves into a plight quite unaided and bear full responsibility for extricating themselves. Yet that hard-headed verdict disregards the desire that parents nearly always have to help their children when they are in trouble; it also fails to take into account the distinct tendency of parents to feel guilty, and even a bit at fault, when things go wrong with their kids.

Though the problems parents experience with adult children can assume a seeming limitless variety of guises, those most prevalent include financial troubles, difficulties with the law, and those associated with sex.

Debbie is 22. Single, attractive, she has a reasonably good job as a bank teller, a position she landed soon after graduating from high school. She lives alone in her own apartment. The rent is $350 per month. Her car payments are $175 per

141

month. She has an extensive wardrobe and she has furnished the apartment with good pieces. She also has charge account debts that, with her rent and car payment, add up to monthly obligations exceeding her take-home pay. She is now being dunned by collection agencies.

Debbie wants her parents to bail her out by lending her enough money to pay off her obligations. The parents are reluctant to do this, first because the amount of money involved is more than they can dig up easily. Second, they do not want to set a precedent because there are other children. Third, and most important, they have watched Debbie's fiscal balancing act for some time, have seen their mild suggestions brushed aside, and have thus developed very little confidence in her ability to manage her affairs to repay the loan.

• • •

Greg, 20, accompanied a group of his friends to a nearby beach. During that afternoon he and two others in the group were arrested for possession and use of drugs. Greg was holding a sufficiently large amount of marijuana to support a felony charge, and one of the others had a small amount of cocaine. All three of them gave evidence of being high when they were apprehended. A scuffle broke out and they were subdued by the officers making the arrest. They were booked and charged with possession, resisting arrest, and assault (one of the officers had been bitten during the excitement). Greg called his parents to inform them of his plight. He wanted to be bailed out and he wanted legal assistance that he could not afford.

The parents went the bail and talked the matter over with Greg before deciding whether or not to get counsel. After being grilled by his parents, Greg admitted that he did in fact have a relatively large quantity of pot and had been dealing small amounts. He believes that the arrest and search were carried out illegally and that there were procedural errors that would result in a dismissal of charges if a competent lawyer were brought in on the case. The parents are extremely angry with and disappointed in Greg, but they do not want him to wind up spending time in the state penitentiary.

Debbie and Greg each present their parents with a problem that permits a number of approaches and varying levels of involvement. Their parents can wash their hands of the matter, they can provide the help desired, they can give aid under specified conditions, they can help the child tap into outside resources. Which option to select depends on the specific complex of factors involved in each instance.

Dealing with Scrapes Effectively

Providing all the help a child wants without attaching conditions or stipulating some sort of payback—either material and/or behavioral—will have little effect on the child's future actions. Thus, lending Debbie the money she needs without imposing restrictions on how she manages her finances will simply not help her to learn to be more responsible in her money management. Engaging legal aid for Greg in the absence of a commitment from him to repay the costs and to clean up his act simply invites him to replay the same scenario.

Crisis situations have a way of blinding individuals to their alternatives. With Greg in the lockup, the first thought is to get him out. Debbie, hounded by creditors and threatened with litigation, needs money now. Or, so it would appear. In urgent, do-something-right-now circumstances like these, options are usually overlooked. In Debbie's case, though she believes she is at the end of her rope, the creditors will wait. All they want is their money and they know they will get it with 20% interest to boot.

Financial counseling is available. Debbie's employer, the bank, maintained just such a service for its employees and she, when told of it, turned to it for help. Organizations that lend money—finance companies, credit unions, savings and loan associations—offer free advice too, but it is wise to be wary of help from individuals or organizations having a financial stake in the decision or the outcome.

The point is that there are public and private organizations that have been established specifically to deal with most of the problems that people get into in our society. Abuse of credit is commonplace in the United States; credit, plastic, is the engine that drives commerce and it is readily available to almost everyone. And, unhappily, many of us find ourselves stretched thin at one time or another. Skilled help and advice with this sort of problem is there for the asking.

So too with violations of the drug laws. In many states, first-time offenders like Greg are often remanded to a "diversion" program with the charge dismissed on completion of a "counseling" course and a successful period of parole. Information on the statutes and typical procedures is usually available through drug counseling and treatment centers that can be found in most large cities and in many smaller communities as well.

Greg's parents did consult with a free drug clinic. They were correctly informed that the charges against Greg would probably be reduced and "diversion" ordered. The clinic also recommended a lawyer, who provided valuable and relatively inexpensive help through the hearings. Greg signed a note for the money his parents advanced and also promised to leave drugs alone; he kept both agreements.

When crises erupt, their suddenness and urgency heighten their apparent gravity. It is important for parents promptly to find out what the problem is and to try to establish what kinds of options exist before making a move. Snap judgments, impulsive decisions reached under stress, too often result in ineffectual decisions and costly mistakes.

Art and Harriet, the parents of 24-year-old Ray, get a telephone call from the father of Ray's girl friend, Sheri. Neither Art nor Harriet likes the girl and they do not approve of Ray's involvement with someone so young. Sheri's father charges that Sheri is pregnant, that Ray is responsible, and that unless he makes it "right" with Sheri, he will be charged with statutory rape and contributing to the delinquency of a minor.

Ray admits that he and Sheri have been having sex and that the child is probably his. He does not want to get married and suggests abortion as an alternative. This solution is rejected by both sets of parents on religious grounds; Sheri also rejects it. She appears to have set up the pregnancy so that she could get married, although Ray certainly has nobody but himself to blame for his problem.

Ray, frightened by the threats, and believing that he has no options, marries the girl. Six months after the child is born Ray separates from Sheri and they are soon divorced. Their divorce is naturally no more tolerable to the parents than abortion would have been.

In this situation all parties failed to consider that there were alternatives besides marriage or abortion—their anger and shame made it impossible for these other possibilities to be entertained. Because of their religious orientation, as well as Sheri's desire to get married and her apparent use of pregnancy as a lever to bring this about, it is likely that none of the options would have been acceptable. But the child might well have been kept, without marriage, or alternatively it might have been borne and offered for adoption.

The traditional solution is "to make it right by the woman" who is seen as—and usually is—the victim.

In this and other instances, however, the "victim" may also be the male. Jerry will pay for his lack of judgment for a long time. Art and Harriet will also pay for being connected to a daughter-in-law they dislike and a grandson they did not want but had to accept. The rest of those involved, not the least of them the child, also cannot escape being affected.

The local Planned Parenthood Association could have helped to spell out options in this instance; facilities are available for the protection and care of unwed mothers; counseling for all of those involved could be secured through Family

Service or other agencies. Though Ray's behavior was heed-less and irresponsible, the penalties for him and for everyone else were much graver than they needed to be.

Getting Help

In talking about various scrapes that adult children can get into, I have stressed taking action or making the decision to get involved only after ascertaining and weighing the alter-natives available. Some of the many helping resources have also been named. Though I cannot possibly catalog all of the unhappy entanglements that children may find themselves trapped in, some measure of assistance or help with every one of them is available—medical advice, legal aid, counseling on every form of dilemma. Directories of helping services are issued periodically in most communities—the Family Service Organization can most likely guide you to such a publication. The key points to remember here are to move promptly but judiciously, not taking hasty or intemperate action, and to seek out and weigh all the alternative courses of action avail-able before proceeding with a specific plan.

PART FOUR

INDIVIDUAL PROBLEMS GROWING OUT OF DIFFERING LIFESTYLES

Children and parents have always disagreed about what constitutes right or proper conduct. Much of the disagreement arises out of an inability or unwillingness to accept, or even to tolerate, one another's "life style."

Lifestyle is a catchall term that stands for the rules of conduct one observes. No two lifestyles are exactly the same, any more than any two individuals are completely alike. However, there are a number of behaviors that grown children exhibit that have always proven especially troublesome for parents to tolerate. These include cohabitation (living together), homosexuality, drug use or abuse, religious or political cult membership, and simple neglect of the parents by the children. This part of *Coping With Your Grown Children* takes up these matters, shows how they concern adult parents, and explains how best they may be addressed—or put to one side.

CHAPTER 12

INDIVIDUAL PROBLEMS OF PARENTS OF ADULT CHILDREN

*Happiness is living long enough
to be a problem to your children.*

Introduction

Adult child–parent problems, as we have seen, fall into two categories—shared or individual. Some of the situations we will be discussing here may upset both parent and child, even though the children unquestionably have the undivided right and responsibility to decide what, if anything, to do about them. Under these conditions of mutual concern, parents may want to conduct themselves as if they were faced with problems like the legal, fiscal, and similar plights described in Chapter 11. In most of the scenarios we will now examine, the child has a clear right to do whatever it is that has been or is being done—the concerned parent is in fact the one with the problem. Parents create these individual problems for themselves in one of two ways: First, by inventing non-existent difficulties, letting the darker side of their imaginations run wild, or second, by intervening in their adult childrens' affairs when they have neither the right nor the responsibility to do so. Clashes over lifestyles are especially prone to such misintepretation and overweening parental concern.

When grown children are untroubled by whatever they are doing, or are striving to manage on their own, the role of the parent becomes more fuzzily defined. Clearly, if a behavior, a lifestyle, is none of the parents' affair, they may not meddle. Yet if the child is behaving in a manner of which the parent disapproves or considers to be wrong, scandalous, or self-destructive, there is an almost irresistible temptation to get involved. Such unwanted and uninvited intervention may then entail especially unhappy consequences—which is a particularly good reason for a hands-off policy.

The succeeding chapters stress the often-overlooked negative consequences of unsolicited intervention, and describe several steps that parents can take either to distance themselves from, or to live more comfortably with, activities and lifestyles they may have great trouble accepting.

Rights of Adults

Parents could spare themselves a great deal of anguish if they accepted the idea that—when children have the right and responsibility to do whatever it is they are doing—they also take clear title to any problems that may ensue. Unhappily, when most parents disapprove of something their children are doing, or are thought to be doing, they tend to intervene, often manufacturing fresh problems for themselves.

These parents too readily forget that having rights frees the individual to make decisions, including bad ones. Adult rights include all of the constitutional guarantees, plus the freedoms established in law or custom. These include freedom of speech and religion, freedom to choose one's own associates, freedom of movement, and, most important, freedom to make one's own life decisions and to bear the consequences, good or bad.

These rights do not apply in those uncommon instances when the individual is not competent to act in his or her own behalf. Judging lack of competence in an adult is a legal matter and is limited to individuals found to be incapable of fending for themselves. Almost all adults are "competent"; almost all adults will, at some time or another, make bad decisions. Real world choices can go sour because of simple mistakes, flawed personal prophecies about the future, erroneous estimates of a situation, omissions or oversights, and rash, impulsive acts.

In the abstract, the principle of the individual's right to decide is clear and simple; in practice, it often becomes much more complicated. Parents, being human, want to have things both ways. They believe in rights, but when the exercise of those rights threatens their own sense of propriety or well-being, they will often attempt to deny them. Freedom for the child, in this instance, amounts to the freedom to do what Mom or Dad approve of. Though most would readily agree that such behavior is overbearing and destructive, parents will defend it, contending that sometimes rights have to be abridged for the "good" (safety, well-being) of the child.

Is an adult child ever "better off" when denied the opportunity to act freely as an adult? Denying the child freedom to choose, to make independent decisions, declares that the training or preparation of the child for adulthood has been neither adequate nor serviceable. Parents bear some of the responsibility for that failure.

Interference with rights also happens for less obvious reasons. Parents often use children, without quite realizing it, in a futile and desperate effort to hold on to their own youth. By keeping a child locked into a dependent relationship, the child remains a child and the parents still youthful. At other times parents use children as extensions of themselves, living their own lives through their children. Thus, the children take on worth, not for what they are so much as for what they represent to others in terms of status or accomplishment.

Observing a child's struggle with a problem is a lot like watching another person trying to unravel a tangle of string. While you watch, your fingers itch to wrest the snarl from the other person and do it yourself. You may even reach out for it and only your own courtesy—or the other person's drawing away from you—will prevent you from snatching it away. It is extremely difficult not to interfere, especially when individuals you care deeply about behave in ways that seem to be inept, ill-considered, and likely to cause them trouble or unhappiness. However, giving in to the temptation to meddle compromises rights that all of us, including our children, possess. In addition, interference may damage the relationship between parent and child or intensify a dependency that, in time, will prove dangerous and crippling to the child. Meddling needs to be resisted at all costs.

Letting Adult Children Be Adults

Adults *do* have indisputable rights. When one set of adults (parents) sets out to deny another set of adults (grown children) their rights, conflict is bound to follow. The conflict usually leads to suffering for the parents because they are in fact powerless to prevent what is occurring. Unhappiness, impaired relationships, and distancing—both physical and emotional—are the payoffs.

Keeping hands off, however difficult, is quite simply the best tactic for middle-aged parents faced with the problem of deciding what to do about children who are either contemplating or already engaging in behavior that seems deplorable to the parents. Given the complex web of emotional ties binding parent and child together, offering that advice is easier than accepting it. Arranging matters so that children experience independence and the opportunity to make significant choices early in life—during childhood and adolescence—is one way of helping them become skilled and confident decision-makers while giving parents valuable practice in not meddling.

Arriving at the point where one really understands and accepts the notion that your adult child has undeniable legal and social rights is crucial to the management of disagreements about lifestyle. It helps if you can come to realize that the child owes you exactly the same freedom to make choices as you owe him or her. You need not approve or endorse whatever the child does, but you must respect his or her right to do it. The child may not accept any of countless features of your lifestyle; he or she should similarly respect your rights. Differences of opinion on even the most troublesome issues need not lead to anger and alienation. That they so often do testifies to the reality that one of the parties—more often than not a parent—has failed to understand and act with due respect for the birthright freedoms that each of us enjoys as an individual, and is meddling rather than trusting.

The ability to let your child go is tied closely to the cultivation of an unconditional regard for the other person, your child, as someone whose rights and responsibilities exactly mirror your own. You raised your children to be independent; to achieve this goal fully you must free them from the outgrown reins of your own authority.

CHAPTER 13

LIFE STYLES AND MEANINGFUL RELATIONSHIPS

> *Dear Abby:*
> *I am heartsick about my daughter. She is 33, attractive, popular,*
> *and well-educated, but to get to the point I am ashamed that*
> *she is living with a man. Whenever I ask her if she plans*
> *to marry him she insists that marriage is not important to her*
> *and she is very happy with things as they are.*
> *(Abby, how can she be happy?)*
> *...I want to die when my friends ask me about her. And I'm a wreck*
> *trying to keep it from the relatives. She was raised in a good Christian*
> *home, went to Sunday school and church regularly, and had good*
> *examples to follow. I don't know where she got these loose,*
> *immoral ideas. How do parents cope with a situation like this?*
> *— Sick at heart*

Introduction

Lifestyles differ widely along socioeconomic, class, age, and ethnic lines, but each is internally consistent. "Straight" middle-aged, middle-class white parents believe and act in certain predictable ways. They can be distinguished from other groups—in dress, hair style, place and type of residence, fiscal habits, opinions on political, moral, and social questions, and language. People in this group follow values

157

rooted in the American past—prudence, industriousness, conservatism (in its broader sense), independence, autonomy, stability, heterosexuality.

At one time this set of values represented something of a norm, but in the past generation the pace of change has quickened, with many different styles becoming important. From an "American plan" we have moved gradually to a smorgasbord of lifestyles, with the followers of each style looking either askance or enviously at the practices of the others.

This social fragmentation of a once nearly monolithic mainstream into a wide variety of lifestyles contributes substantially to conflict between parents and children—despite our conviction that our children should have the right to select a way of life that suits themselves. The multiplicity of styles involves many different assumptions and rules of conduct; it is disagreement over these basic precepts that carries the seeds of our discord.

Of all the ways in which parents' and childrens' lifestyles can differ, those arising from disagreements about material values and sexual mores are responsible for the most severe misunderstandings.

Material Values

The depression of the 1930s shaped today's middle-aged generation, conditioning it to seek security first, to look to the future. That generation's children, however, have grown up in an era of relatively steady economic growth and prosperity, and so have avoided falling into the depression mentality of their parents.

Fred remembers the depression vividly because it cheated him out of a lot of things. With his father unemployed, he had started working at various kinds of jobs as soon as he could simply to help the family survive. He had worked all during grade and high school; on graduation, he had been lucky enough to find a full-time job in a machine shop. He is still employed there as a machinist. He and his wife, Irma, have lived carefully, saved, bought property, and made other blue chip investments so that they are now extremely well-off. But Fred feels that he never really had a childhood.

He worries that his only child, Eric, will never have an adulthood. Eric graduated from high school and then went to college for a time. He dropped out, served in the Army, came back, found a job, worked at it for a while, quit it, went to another job, and then another. He shares an old house with a miscellaneous and continually changing group of house-mates, male and female. He seems to have enough to get by on, enjoys life, has many friends, and is on good terms with Fred and Irma. Fred does not approve of Eric's easy-come, easy-go approach to life and he worries that Eric is not planning adequately for the future. He tries to talk to Eric about it because he is genuinely concerned, but Eric simply shrugs him off, calling him a "worry wart" and telling him that he can always find something to do.

In the light of his own harsh experiences with real hardship, it is easy to understand Fred's concern and his attempts to urge Eric into showing more concern for his future. Eric has no understanding of his father's early experiences and of the impact of the depression. It is extremely difficult for him or anyone else to imagine the feelings of insecurity and dread that Fred experienced. These feelings have followed him and many of his generation throughout their lives.

Fred knows only one way of dealing with economic uncertainty and it has worked well for him. Reasoning from his own experience, he believes that Eric should follow his example. However, Eric, who likes and respects his father, is not at all attracted to a life that revolves around self-denial and the threat of scarcity. He prefers to take his chances.

Though Fred has not let his concern about Eric and Eric's approach to life reach the point where it overrides everything else, it does gnaw at him. He would be more content if he could simply accept Eric's freedom to choose his own way of life. It is not, after all, illegal, and it is pleasant and congenial, even though it is not "secure" in Fred's view. Moreover, Fred simply cannot understand, and feels upset by, Eric's blithe disregard for material values. Eric drives an old wreck of a car; he doesn't carry insurance on it. He owns few things beyond his clothes. He does not like or use banks and operates mainly out of his pocket, buying what he needs when he needs it and paying cash for it. When he doesn't have enough cash, he bides his time. Fred can't understand Eric's not wanting good or "nice" things, not having resources on hand for that "rainy day," not even having or wanting a savings account. Yet he still strives vainly to convert Eric to his views. It would be easier on him—and on Eric—if he recognized that Eric had made a free choice of lifestyle to which he is eminently entitled.

Though Fred experiences a persistent low level of unhappiness about Eric's improvident, carefree style and does what little he can to turn it around, Eric is untroubled by Fred's attempts to convert him. The relationship, despite Fred's concern and his attempts to manage Eric's life, is warm and durable. Fred is the one with the problem and it grows out of his unwillingness to permit Eric to have matters his own way. Things will improve for Fred when he honestly realizes that Eric is free to live his own life and begins looking at all of the affirmative qualities that Eric displays. But despite all, they manage to get along fine.

Sexual Mores

Molly and Jim represent a different problem altogether.

Molly is just twenty-two. She and Jim have been living together for just over two years, although Molly's parents, Hank and Jane, have known of it for only the past year. Molly and Jim entered into the liaison after discussing it fully and making an "agreement" that spells out their rights and obligations.

Molly hesitated about telling her parents because she knew that they strongly disapprove of sex outside of marriage and vehemently condemn "shacking up," which is how they refer to Molly and Jim's arrangement. However, she felt obliged to inform her parents and, in spite of her misgivings, did so.

Her worst fears were realized. Her mother became hysterical with grief and self-reproach. Her father's reaction was worse. "Who is it?" he asked. (Neither parent had met Jim.)

Molly tried to tell him about Jim and their agreement and their feelings for one another. Hank listened through it all and had the last word. "Don't ever bring that son-of-a-bitch around here," he said.

Molly obeyed. She has not seen or talked to her father since. She phones her mother periodically at times when she knows her father is not at home and notices that her mother is glad to hear from her. Recently her mother has called her, apparently willing to run the risk of speaking with Jim. But her father remains intransigent and, according to her mother, grows more bitter and angry as the period of separation lengthens. Molly believes strongly that she has the right to live her life on her own terms. She also believes that it is up to her father to initiate any steps in the direction of reconciliation, convinced that there can be no improvement until he is ready to change.

I have not mentioned Jim's parents because they accept and support the arrangement. Opposition to these kinds of "meaningful relationships," whatever the euphemism—cohabitation, roommate, partnership, liaison and so on—will more likely occur in the family of the woman, although that is somewhat tempered by ethnic and class differences. In this case Jim's parents are extremely fond of Molly and see that the relationship is solid and will probably endure.

Molly's father, angry and bitterly disapproving, owns this problem. His solution—and it would only be a partial one at that because he is not the sort of person to let bygones be bygones—would be for Molly to break up with Jim. It is not especially likely that Molly's marrying Jim would help matters much—the father is carrying too great a grudge to hope that even a strained and uneasy truce might result.

And Molly's mother, though she disapproves of the affair, has her own problem. She has come to the point where she can accept matters as they are and wants to reestablish more normal relationships with Molly, knowing that this will require contact and communication with Jim. She is willing to do this, but her husband not only refuses to consider it, he forbids her to have anything to do with Jim. Her resentment of his stubbornness and his authoritarianism is growing, and it was this feeling of helpless anger that brought her to me for help.

The incidence of premarital cohabitation has increased dramatically in the past twenty years and certainly involves a substantial proportion of young adults. Recent polls reveal that fewer than half of twenty-one year olds disapprove of such arrangements; however, three quarters of the fifty and older generation condemn cohabitation and over half of them disapprove of any premarital sexual activity at all. With the generations so deeply divided in their opinions about these volatile matters, intense disagreements result. Even with parents who are less inclined to stick to traditional views about what is proper, cohabitation often comes as a shock.

Notwithstanding parental feelings and opinions, consenting adults do have the right to enter into relationships, meaningful or not. In some states, living together for a period of time and under specified conditions has in fact been given legal recognition tantamout to marriage. Court decisions have found that rights do inhere in such relationships even though no formal written contract—marital or otherwise—was entered into.

Though adult children may feel conflict and guilt about these relationships, these feelings more often arise out from the reactions the parents have and the knowledge that the parents will try to interfere with or control their actions, even when they have no right to do so. The child runs the risk of parental displeasure, but it is not the responsibility of the child to please the parent. Rather, the parent must recognize and accept the right of the child to make decisions and, having made them, to live with them and their consequences.

The Lifestyle Boom

The emergence of a wide variety of lifestyles owes much to the evolution of a distinctive youth culture and the social movements of the 60s and early 70s. In fact, individuals seem to proceed through different styles as their personal circumstances change; the flower children of the sixties have become the upscale baby boomers of the eighties.

That a number of conflicting lifestyles can coexist also owes much to the breakdown of the traditional WASP values and their replacement with a range of alternatives that accord work, conservatism, and "morality" lesser importance. This breakdown, as noted in Chapter 2, has its roots in the rapid and pervasive technological change that has so deeply touched most aspects of American life since World War II.

Paradoxically, some young adults are trying to live a more austere, reclusive life, and thus to enter into what has been called the "postindustrial" society. They hold radically different views about materialism, about the durability and permanence of relationships, about economic, social, and political institutions. The asceticism implicit in this attitude toward life sometimes baffles middle-aged parents.

Another source of dissension lies in the radical change in sexual proprieties that has occurred. This development has been greatly facilitated by medical advances that have made the prevention or termination of pregnancies simple and safe. With birth control measures readily accessible and with abortion a common recourse in the event of unwanted or unplanned pregnancy, the social and psychological taboos on premarital sexual activity have eased dramatically.

Though there are many other factors that contribute to this turnabout, the major points of difference between parents and children are found mainly in the rejection (or, at least, the denial of relevance) of many of the most deeply held attitudes, values, and mores of the parents, and the inability of the parents to recognize that their children have the right to reject them, however wrong the parents may view this rejection to be.

Getting Help

To profit from those sources of help that are readily available, middle-aged parents who find themselves unhappy and distressed over a conflict in lifestyles must first be able to admit that an admissable alternative point of view is at least possible. Without this, seeking help would be a waste of time. After all, when there is a steadfast belief that one is in the right, the search for help amounts to nothing more than a quest for support for one's own cherished position.

At the outset, troubled parents should at least take stock of the reasons for their unhappiness. Are they rooted in what the child is actually doing? Do the parents want to understand or tolerate the child's actions, even though they cannot? Do they find it quite impossible to express their feelings about the child's behavior and feel frustrated and helpless at this inability?

If the problem amounts to a pure case of unhappiness with the child's behavior, the parents must simply tell the child. This can, and should, be done directly and openly—without creating a scene. Parents should concentrate on expressing their own feelings and concerns, and steer clear of criticizing or reproaching the child since that will almost certainly prove counterproductive.

When the parent is unable to be direct or open, getting outside help may break the impasse. Group sessions conducted expressly for middle-aged persons often prove useful and, if they are being offered in your community, can be readily found by following the procedures outlined in Chapter 20. In some instances, individual treatment may be called for—or preferred. Where and what to look for in this eventuality are also outlined there.

CHAPTER 14

GAY OR LESBIAN CHILDREN

Introduction

The number of homosexuals in the United States is estimated at five to ten percent of the population—somewhere
between 12 and 25 million individuals. According to Kinsey,
one-third of the population has had at least one homosexual
encounter. Despite the prevalence of homosexuality, much of
the general public has remained stubbornly unenlightened
about, and opposed to, homosexuality and homosexual behavior. In the past few years, however, there has been a
growing awareness of the wide existence of homosexuality.
This has come about because of the increasing willingness of

individuals who prefer homosexual lifestyles to "come out"—
to permit their sexual preferences to be publicly known.

This disposition to openness—to an honest, direct, and
candid assertion of sexual orientation and preference—has
led some to conclude wrongly that homosexuality was becoming more common. It has also had some additional consequences. First, there was initially a somewhat greater willingness to accept homosexuality as a style of life; this acceptance
has probably been withdrawn to an extent during the past few
years with the outbreak of Acquired Immune Deficiency Syndrome, or AIDS. This condition, apparently virus-borne,
causes a breakdown in the body's defense mechanisms and
renders its victims vulnerable to other fatal diseases. AIDS,
though showing recent signs that it is spreading to other
groups in the population, is still largely found in homosexual
males and intravenous drug users.

The appearance of AIDS, its rapid spread, and its deadli-
ness have intensified the negative feelings that many individuals bear toward homosexuals and have fueled attempts both
to safeguard and to sharply curtail the human rights of AIDS
victims. The fear that the disease provokes, much of it irrational and without basis in fact, invites impulsive and often
destructive reactions.

Second, it has been the cause of great unhappiness or distress in many parents who learn about homosexuality in their
own children. When the general climate of public opinion
was even less prone to accept homosexuality, there was a cor-
respondingly greater tendency for homosexuals to keep their
sexual orientation hidden. As a consequence parents, whatever their suspicions, did not have to confront the fact of
homosexuality in their children directly.

No area of grown-child behavior is likely to prove more
unsettling to a parent than learning that the child is homosexual—gay or lesbian. And here, especially, the parents are
prone to view that outcome as evidence of their failure as

parents. This tendency to assume blame may be especially tempting because of the religious proscriptions attached to homosexuality and the negative values and sanctions that accompany it. Certainly, almost all parents expect that their children will be heterosexual and bring them up with that idea in mind. There is no evidence at all to suggest that parents are instrumental in inducing homosexual behavior; the gravity that parents attach to the discovery has to do with the pre-existing attitudes, largely negative, that parents bring to homosexuality.

Homosexuality also represents a problem for the child, obviously so in a society that is predominantly and assertively heterosexual. However, the problems of the child and of the parent are not usually complementary. The homosexual is most often concerned about disclosure and the kinds of personal, economic, and social consequences it will have. These are to be balanced against the decision to keep silent and thus to experience the feelings of self-loathing, shame, and guilt that usually accompany that choice.

The parents are also concerned about disclosure and the condemnation or pity that will accrue to them and to their child because of it. Both parties are in a bad place.

Larry is in his mid-thirties. A bit above average height and somewhat overweight, he is fussy about his appearance. He speaks carefully, somewhat pedantically, in a pleasant, deep voice. He has been living with his male lover, to whom he refers as his spouse, for ten years. They are both sober, conservative individuals who lead responsible, orderly, and, in many respects, humdrum lives.

Larry does not know how he became gay. As early as he can remember he was attracted to boys or men rather than to girls or women. Larry grew up in a midwest city in a neighborhood that was beginning to be occupied by black families and he recalls with amusement his parents' warnings not to become involved with black girls.

Larry developed a keen interest in religion. He made good grades in high school and won a scholarship to a nearby college that had a program in religious studies. While at college he had his first homosexual experience with another student, a serious and important affair that ended when the partner dropped out of school.

Fully aware of his orientation and troubled by it, Larry tried psychotherapy, which failed to help him either to accept his homosexuality or to develop heterosexual alternatives. He graduated from college with high grades and, prior to graduation, applied for admission to a seminary to train for the ministry. By now he admitted his homosexuality openly and disclosed it on his application for admission to the theological school. The application was rejected.

Larry had also told his mother about his homosexuality. His father had died while Larry was an undergraduate and had not been aware that Larry was gay. Larry's mother did not seem to grasp what Larry was trying to tell her and has clung to this attitude of blank incomprehension. Larry, at first angered by his mother's stubborn refusal or inability to accept what he was telling her, tried to break through this defense because he wanted her to know and understand his situation. He failed, gave up trying, and now wryly accepts his mother's obtuseness. But he comments that they are about as close as strangers sharing the same pair of seats on a bus. He is relieved that she has remained in the midwest so that their stilted visits are rare and brief.

Larry has come to terms with his situation. So, in her way, has his mother by blocking out or not even grasping what she has been told. The understanding of homosexuality may in some individual instances be so sketchy that there is no way of comprehending or assimilating the idea; what is inconceivable, unimaginable, can be put out of mind.

In this case, there is no problem for either the mother or Larry. Larry is matter-of-fact about his sexual orientation, secure in his stable relationship, able to deal with any troubles that may grow out of it.

Mother doesn't recognize a problem. Though she views Larry in false terms—still asking him, periodically, if he has any plans or prospects about marriage—she is not bothered by what she cannot see. Though her denial is in some sense bizarre, it spares her anguish.

Larry's mother's response is one way of dealing with a child's homosexuality. The most common response of parents is a massive outpouring of self-blame and guilt. In some parents, there is an angry and punitive reaction; other parents use the face-saving device of believing that the child is using homosexuality as a means of getting back at them, of hurting them in the cruelest way imaginable.

"Treating" Homosexuality

Ordinary people, unlike mental health specialists, are inclined to regard homosexuality as aberrant or "sick." When this attitude is held by parents, as it often is, the first move is to try to direct the child into psychotherapy. Psychotherapy has had scant success in reorienting gays or lesbians sexually. It may be quite helpful in assisting homosexual persons to resolve their feelings about their lifestyle, and can aid the parents in handling the self-blame, guilt, anxiety, or the sense of failure that often accompanies the discovery of a child's homosexuality. But psychotherapy will not change sexual preference. Shirley's experience is typical.

Shirley, an only child, grew up in comfortable circumstances. Extremely bright, attractive, and popular, she made outstanding grades in high school and was accepted at a prestigious university. Though she had dated in high school she had never felt particularly comfortable in that sort of relationship with boys—somehow she felt in competition with them and, certainly, her skill at sports and her daring, amounting to foolhardiness, on skis or motorcycles or in racing sports cars made the competition real.

She became engaged while at the university and lived with her fiancé for the last year there, but the relationship was not particularly satisfying to her, sexually or otherwise, because she and her fiance "were too much alike." The couple broke up just about the time she graduated.

She returned to her home town and enrolled for graduate study at the university there. She found part-time work and her parents kept her on an allowance so that she was able to get along comfortably. She continued in her competitive activities, particularly skiing, but they came to an end when she took a bad fall and broke her leg. She was hospitalized for weeks and on crutches for several months. During that time she came to know another woman, a graduate student who chauffered her to and from classes and with whom, eventually, she established a lesbian relationship.

She felt compelled to tell her parents and did this one evening, just at the end of dinner. It was an uncomfortable scene since Shirley, not knowing exactly how to proceed, blurted out, "Mother...Dad...I think I should tell you, I think you have the right to know that I'm a...a lesbian."

The parents were quite thunderstruck and a long silence followed. It was finally broken when the mother started weeping. Shirley went to comfort her. The mother recoiled. "Don't touch me," she commanded. "I can't stand it. Oh, God, what's happened to you? What's become of you?"

Shirley's father, silent until then, ashen, made his contribution. "You've got to get help. We can't have this." The attitudes of the parents were so unyielding that, against her better judgment, Shirley agreed to see a psychiatrist. She met with the therapist twice a week for almost a year but, as Shirley tells it, "She spent all of her time trying to find out what it was in my background that had turned me on to women and we never got anywhere. I didn't feel any different after a year except that I was tired of talking to her and it was costing a lot of money. So I told her that I wasn't going to see her any more and I told my parents that it was just wasting time and throwing money away; that I didn't feel any different."

By that time the parents had been able to take stock of the situation, and though they by no means supported the idea, they were now able to tolerate it. Shirley left home and she and her lover moved into an apartment. Both of them work full-time and have carved out a life for themselves in the community. Shirley's active, public, and militant espousal of gay and lesbian rights has not pleased the parents, who would prefer that she keep a low profile, but her lifestyle has not affected theirs. They have met and, after some initial awkwardness and reserve, have come to like and accept Shirley's lover. They will probably never be fully comfortable with Shirley's choice, but they have come to the point where they can live with it and not feel that Shirley is "sick."

Shirley was luckier than some because it only took her a relatively short time to learn that the situation could not be "straightened out" psychotherapeutically. She therefore felt free not to allow herself to persist in an uncomfortable and unproductive course of treatment.

Nobody fully understands the causes, the roots of homosexuality. Even if the causes were understood, the means available would seem to be largely ineffectual in bringing about changes in sexual orientation. Thus, the task of both the parent and the child finding themselves in this situation is to come to the best terms possible with it.

The "best terms possible" will of course vary with the individuals concerned. In extreme cases, the attitudes of parents toward homosexuality are so harsh and condemnatory that the only sensible course to follow is for parents and child to break — certainly an unhappy and destructive solution, but the best one available.

Larry and Shirley have found relatively satisfactory resolutions of a common dilemma in our society. Solutions are not always so easily achieved however, because the behavior of either the child or parent can be extreme, overreactive, intransigent, bizarre. For a more thorough discussion of these difficult problems, Charles Silverstein's book, *A Family Mat-*

ter: A parent's guide to homosexuality, is warmly recommended. It gives a complete and rounded picture that is sympathetic to both parent and child. His list of "Dos" and "Don'ts" for parents is particularly valuable.

Origins

Theories of personality development advance a variety of different reasons to account for homosexuality. They are mainly speculative, rife with contradictions, and offer little persuasive evidence to explain the phenomenon. At this stage nobody knows what causes homosexuality. The popular tendency to blame homosexuality on malparenting does not receive any support from the data; this hypothesis is contradicted by the unexplained and inconsistent emergence of homosexuality in milieus that differ ethically, socially, economically, or religiously. Homosexuality is encountered in families varying in every imaginable way; single-parent families, families following authoritarian, democratic, or laissez-faire methods of child-rearing, families with many children, single-child families, and so on.

In commenting on their homosexuality, many men and women have reported that they were aware of their tendencies and preferences at a very early age and most of them believe that the disposition is fully formed by the age of five years.

There is no evidence to justify the indictment of parents and no valid reason for the overwhelming parental tendency to assume responsibility for homosexuality found in their children. In studies of animals, the failure of heterosexual tendencies to emerge seems to be linked to morbid environmental factors—catastrophic overcrowding and the like—but this does not seem to extend to human experience or conditions.

Getting Help

Despite official stands by both the American Psychiatric and Psychological Associations—which rule that it is not an "illness"—homosexuality is often considered "deviant." A first response, as we have noted, is often to enter the child into some form of therapy that usually fails to change the sexual orientation.

Therapy does have its place, however, both for homosexuals and their parents. Psychotherapy is useful in aiding individuals to accept and understand things as they are, whether in the homosexual child or in the guilt and blame-wracked parent. In those cases in which there is conflict, therapy may aid in its resolution; such distressing side reactions as depression may also respond to treatment.

Since discovery that a child is homosexual often proves devastating for parents, it is important to attempt to understand the nature of the problem. For those parents needing help with their feelings, support groups composed of the parents of gay children have proved to be particularly effective. The standard reactions of parents will surface in such gatherings, and are generally dealt with in compassionate and constructive ways. Parents who attend learn that there are other parents who are experiencing the same kinds of problems as they are. They see how these other individuals deal with their feelings, learn how to relate to their children, and gradually find their way to a position that understands and tolerates their child's choices. There is almost certainly nothing that anyone can do to change the underlying state of affairs—but what can be changed are the attitudes toward it.

CHAPTER 15

CULT MEMBERSHIPS

All religions must be tolerated...
for...every man must get to heaven his own way.

Introduction

The United States has always been hospitable to social fads and experiments. Religious movements, especially, have flourished in an environment that, from its beginnings, provided a haven from religious persecution and made religious freedom a basic tenet. Every era in the history of the country has been marked by the appearance, the spread, and the decline of various religious and other cults and movements.

Usually founded and headed by charismatic leaders, these movements have always promised much—and have always demanded much in return. Aimee Semple McPherson only wanted to hear the rustle of paper when the collection plate went around; Oral Roberts declared God came to him saying Oral must raise $8 million or he would be "called home." Some founders and leaders of movements have been exposed as nothing more than charlatans who used religion as a means of bilking their followers.

What Forms Do Cults Take?

Not all religious movements are evangelistic or Christian; other forms of religious and spiritual expression have enjoyed widespread if brief periods of popularity. Eastern religions have recently drawn disciples, and spiritual leaders such as Maharishi Mahesh Yogi have attracted bands of followers.

The tenets of Islam have proved an important force in the black community in recent years; two strong leaders—Malcolm X and Elijah Muhammed—have already come and gone. Most influential figures from the black community have had well-established religious roots, notably Dr. Martin Luther King, Jr. and the Reverend Jesse Jackson.

Examples of proselytizing religious movements active in recent years include the "Hare Krishna," whose top-knotted, saffron-robed circles of chanting panhandlers were once a familiar sight; the Unification Church, a fundamentalist Christian sect whose followers are called "Moonies" after the founder of the sect, the Reverend Sun Young Moon; and the late L. Ron Hubbard's Church of Scientology.

Not all movements are short-lived. The Church of Jesus Christ of Latter Day Saints began as a small cult under the charismatic Joseph Smith and had to flee westward several times to escape persecution. It has become a respected, powerful, and conservative force in contemporary religious life.

And not all movements are religious. Communes (in themselves not an innovation since the history of the country is rife with communal groups and social experiments of astonishing and sometimes scandalous variety) consisting of individuals who banded together intentionally or who followed a leader to, generally, a rural setting where they could pursue a simpler, more pastoral lifestyle have been common.

Movements and fads that demand a quasireligious commitment were always around—various dietary regimens, jogging, meditation, astrology, psychism, Couéism, and so on.

The religious movements have had one thing in common: the demand for total commitment to the tenets of the faith. This is as true today as it has been in the past. If there is any change, it seems to be away from a heavy emphasis on ever-lasting rewards with more attention now being paid to achieving satisfaction, a sense of peace, social justice, or leading a responsible existence now.

Less important, but still part of the scene and very much objects of media scrutiny, have been the political movements that have also demanded a heavy ideological investment. Those associated with the New Left had a brief flurry of popularity during the sixties and seventies. Small militant radical groups sprang up. They had little aggregate impact, but they did command the undivided loyalty of groups of followers located mainly on college campuses. They also managed to attract a disproportionate (to their size and influence) amount of attention from the media. The various radical left groups have largely faded from the scene, although their criticisms of aspects of the political, economic, and social systems did command attention for a time and there are still some followers to be found.

More recently there has been an outcropping of militant conservative groups. These small bands espouse a variety of views; the most prominent ones are the paramilitary survivalists whose energies are directed to devising and putting into place strategies and means for surviving a nuclear holocaust. Others are, in effect, antigovernment protestors who reject and resist the right of the government to regulate their lives—from levying taxes to requiring driver's licenses. Still others espouse any of a raft of neo-Nazi or other racist views. These groups are secretive, monolithic, tightly disciplined, and ideologically rigid. Narrow self-interest and a callous disregard for others seem to be among their more conspicuous features.

Cults, Children, and Parents

Children who get caught up in something as demanding, alienating, and all-encompassing as conversion to one or another of these cults often constitute a particularly anguishing problem for their parents, partly because the parents reject the tenets of the movement and partly because there is often a flavor of repression or "brainwashing" attached to the process of recruitment.

Bob and his wife, Helen, live in an ashram, a place for meditation and contemplation in Los Angeles. Bob has been there for almost ten years; Helen a bit less than that. Twice they have journeyed to India to sit with the founder and spiritual leader of the sect.

Their modest living costs—$200 per month for the two of them—are borne by Bob's father, who has said he will support Bob and Helen so long as he is able. The other parents involved—Helen's mother and father and Bob's mother—bitterly resent this generosity. They characterize it as pure waste and as counterproductive, in that it permits the young people to persist in their incomprehensible activities and their separation from their parents. All three of them believe that they have lost their children to a charlatan who has victimized a number of young people and uses their contributions for his own selfish purposes. They reason that if the monthly contribution were stopped, Bob and Helen would have to drop out of the ashram and would then come back to them. They see the children periodically. They are free to visit the ashram, and Bob and Helen do return for holidays if someone sends them plane tickets, but the parents feel as if they are in the presence of strangers, of people they don't know or understand. They mourn the loss of their children and they want them back, as they once were.

The disagreement that had smoldered for years came to a head during a particularly bitter quarrel between Bob's parents. Such grave accusations were hurled and such intense feelings of animosity were expressed—mainly by the mother —that after things cooled off a bit they realized that their marriage itself must be on very shaky ground because of the issue. They then sought counseling in order to try and work matters out.

Though it is difficult to stand by and watch Bob and Helen's seeming flight from life, it is even more trying for parents to know that a child has adopted a style of living and a set of beliefs that not only fly in the face of what one accepts, but appears weird or crazed to most other people.

A child devoted to inner search and the quest for harmony, such as Bob or Helen, may or may not be a problem. But a militant Christian who regards parents as lost sinners and aggressively seeks their redemption can be a nearly intolerable burden to shoulder.

Sharon had a religious experience while attending junior college—an inexplicable feeling of insight and revelation that, as she put it, "led me to Christ." Her parents and brothers and sisters are not especially religious, although they live responsible, decent lives. Sharon now considers the rest of her family to be unredeemed sinners who, unless they are reborn in Christ, are condemned to eternal punishment in the afterlife. Since she cares for her parents, she tries unrelentingly to bring about their conversion. The parents resent her unflagging attempts to intercede in their affairs. Though Sharon lives independently, she visits her parents' home often, where she spends much of her time praying and entreating them to join her in seeking spiritual guidance and revelation.

With Sharon growing more insistent and more preoccupied with their graceless state, the parents became alarmed at her actions and sought advice on what to do. They began to think that Sharon had lost her judgment, her ability to function competently, and they considered the advisability of having her declared "incompetent," even though this step would cause them no less grief and pain than is aroused by Sharon's excess of pious zeal.

Though the children in both of the instances described above have made extreme choices, it is necessary to remember that the decisions are their own to make, just as Bob's father's election to underwrite Bob and Helen's life is also mainly his to make. The decision to follow some ideal—or belief or cause or idol—that displeases the parents, that no longer locates them centrally in the lives and well-being of their children, is hard to accept. Children do, after all, leave home, and their loyalties do shift, but when they leave with a vengeance and when they adopt patterns or ideas that are not only strange, but are viewed with suspicion, amusement, or downright contempt by the rest of society, the shock to the parents can be especially severe. Yet life itself often seems an endless run of bad decisions. They are an inescapable part of the fabric of life in a free society, and people can be protected from their "mistakes" only by a wholesale undermining of the premises on which such a free society rests.

One can argue that Bob and Helen and Sharon each have "problems"—that they are not "normal." Perhaps so. Sharon, in her own way, displays precisely the same kind of overbearing, authoritarian, overprotective behavior that many parents are prone to. And she shows even less respect for her own parents' rights than they do for hers. Her motives, which focus on the welfare of the parents, are no less altruistic than theirs. In this instance, two sets of wrongs add up to a hefty disregard for individual rights.

There is no single way in which children are caught up in movements, cults, religious sects. Most never get involved at all. Those who do are probably trying to escape from something in their lives that they find intolerable. The precipitating cause may be a lack of direction, the shattering of ideals, an absence of and the need for certainty and direction, the vision of escape from poverty or discrimination, a need to express anger, to aggrandize self, to scapegoat, and so on. Involvement with any of a wide range of activities—joining a movement, cult, or community, for instance—frees the individual from existing connections. Stress or overload may impel these radical redirections or withdrawals. The decision to escape or to attack the problem head-on is (regardless of the social value the chosen solution carries) honest. Though it may distress, sadden, or alienate parents, almost any nontrivial action or step that children may take carries these risks.

About Alienation, Estrangement, and Ethics

Involvement with a cult is a way of addressing failure in the individual or in society—a step in the search for inner harmony, personal security, or a more nearly perfect world. Involvement may be brief, or enduring—and the result of the experience may or may not reconcile the individual to whatever it was that prompted the decision. Discontent, either with the dominant values of the society or with oneself, give impetus to the decision to affiliate.

Affiliation demands more than a simple Pledge of Allegiance. It calls for the replacement of commitments, a transfer of loyalties. It requires work and obedience, and it may entail (as in the case of the Unification Church) undergoing an intensive, high-pressure indoctrination that conditions (some say "programs") the acolyte to the dogma and the demands of the cult. To forge new bonds, the preexisting connections must be severed and this is best done by highlighting the inadequacy, decadence, or wickedness of one's past. Dissatisfaction and the search for a better way underlies cult involvement. (This should not be taken as either apology for or acceptance of the cynically manipulative, self-serving, and right-denying activities of which some movements are guilty.) Recruitment activities are concentrated in environments where the inhabitants are likely to be unhappy with themselves or their lot. Breaking or weakening the ties can be accomplished fairly readily; bitter estrangement from parents often follows.

Getting Help

When an adult child becomes deeply involved with a cult or religious movement, the parents have little or no recourse. In some instances parents have resorted to hiring "deprogrammers," but that tactic has been found by the courts to violate the individual rights of the children to make such choices.

The main options for parents are first, to satisfy themselves that the activity itself is not illegal and the child is not being defrauded or otherwise victimized. Visiting the child, or otherwise finding out as much as possible about what goes on and what obligations he or she has within the movement, is certainly important. If it appears that there are questionable, and possibly illegal, activities, steps can be initiated by making inquiries or filing a complaint through appropriate legal channels.

After discovering as much as possible about what their child is involved with, and seeing to it that the child is not being victimized, the parents may well need help in arriving at a clear understanding that the child has an absolute right to follow the path he or she has chosen. Similarly, they may need help in working through their own feelings of distress at the child's decision. A minister, priest, or other religious figure can often help in this effort. Religious groups are found among the extracurricular organizations on campus at most colleges. Some of them will have full or part-time directors who are familiar with this sort of problem, who know the ethical issues involved, and who have been trained as counselors. If such consultation is not feasible, any of the counseling sources listed in the final chapter might also be consulted.

CHAPTER 16

ABUSE OF SUBSTANCES

Wine is a mocker; strong drink is raging.

Introduction

Addiction to, dependency on, or abuse of drugs is on the rise at all levels of American society. Though parents are more inclined to be concerned about substances like cocaine, heroin, or marijuana, alcohol represents the gravest problem, with prescription or over-the-counter drugs the next most serious threat to the well-being of millions of Americans.

The extent and severity of the alcohol abuse problem is astounding. Seventy-one percent of a sample of adults interviewed by the Gallup organization in 1984 believed that drinking was a very serious problem. In another survey, 84% of respondents favored a required school course on the effects of alcohol and drugs. Teen-agers themselves name alcohol as one of the three most serious problems facing their generation, and substantial proportions of teenage drinkers acknowledge occasionally drinking to excess. Nearly one-quarter of a sample of adults admitted that liquor had been a cause of trouble in the family; this percentage is double that reported only two decades earlier, in 1966.

The percentage of individuals who drink has shown a steady increase and now stands at 67% of all adults; the figures are higher for men, younger persons, and individuals in the higher income brackets.

The social and economic costs of alcohol abuse are staggering; when the effects of drugs are thrown in, the total amounts to what is likely the country's most serious and stubborn domestic problem.

The Consequences of Substance Abuse

Experts do not agree on what constitutes safe levels of drug or alcohol consumption. For some drugs, such as the morphine derivatives, probably no "safe" level of use exists. A number of authorities believe that alcohol in limited quantities, under specified conditions of ingestion, has beneficial results. Yet, in many individual instances, even taking a very small amount of alcohol brings about radical changes in personality and behavior. The long-term effects of alcohol are known to be physically and psychologically harmful; those of some drugs in common if illegal use, like marijuana, remain open to question, although evidence of their dangers is beginning to pile up.

Prescription drugs, especially the mood-altering ones aimed at the conditions that alcohol or "dope" address—building self-confidence, masking or deadening pain, lessening feelings of anxiety or depression, and so on—often have addictive properties. Many of them are also marked by the ability of the user to develop a tolerance for the substance. Consequently, increasing dosages are required if the drug is to remain effective. This feature carries substantial additional dangers, either from overdosing or having two drugs—for example, alcohol and barbiturates—combine lethally.

Drug abuse has malign short- and long-term physical and psychological effects. In the short run, impairment of judgment and disturbance of motor coordination are commonplace; alcohol is a factor in one-half of the approximately 40,000 annual traffic fatalities in the United States. Over a period of time, drug abuse may damage vascular, adrenal, and neurological systems substantially and irreversibly. It may permanently disrupt higher functions, such as patterns and rhythms of sleep, and interfere with immediate and remote memory functions. The social cost, when measured in time lost from or impaired efficiency at work, and the stress in family relationships is incalculable. The annual direct cost to governments in dealing with the problem of public intoxication—from arrest, to the drunk tank, to maintaining detoxification centers and other services addressed to the abuse of all manner of substances—adds up to billions of dollars.

Drug abuse reaches into all levels of society, from the neonate born with a heroin habit acquired from a junkie mother, to the octogenarian who downs 60 grains of aspirin a day just to dull some of the aches and pains associated with old age. It is especially prevalent among young adults, in whom the incidence and excessive use of most kinds of drugs is higher than for other age groups in the population.

> Elena started drinking when she was a sophomore in high school, 12 years ago. When she got home from school she would help herself to a couple of shots from her father's half gallon of cheap vodka. The father had a drinking problem, although he wouldn't acknowledge it. "Never missed a day on the job," he would boast, and that was true. And he stayed out of trouble on the highways by doing all of his drinking at home, making himself more or less senseless by ten in the evening when he would fall into a stuporous, drunken sleep. He had died suddenly four years earlier from complications brought on by his drinking.

Elena graduated from high school and managed to find work, but her drinking affected her job performance and she was let go. She drifted from one marginal job to another, but never held on to one for very long. She has not worked for over four years now and lives on general assistance, supplemented by money which she earns caring for children. A small allowance from her mother helps with the rent. Her mother is acutely aware of Elena's problem and continually nags her to take some action to break the habit. Elena denies that she drinks too much; she also declares that she can quit any time she wants to.

Frustrated because she could not persuade Elena that she had a problem that needed to be acted on, the mother came to me for advice. She expressed concern about the gravity of Elena's problem—at least a fifth of vodka a day, starting before breakfast and continuing until bedtime—and she is worried about what Elena will do, how she will manage when she, the mother, is gone.

Bill, when I first got to know him, had just been released from the state penitentiary after doing five years for a series of armed robberies. He looked like the quintessential biker.

Bill owed many of his problems to drug abuse, combining incredible quantities and mixtures of drugs. While on drugs, but at other times, too, he engaged in various kinds of rebellious and unlawful behavior that constantly had him in trouble with the police. Aside from brief jail stays, intervention from his parents—both of them teachers—kept him out of deep trouble with the law. One night, however, he and a friend got "loaded" and held up a liquor store. They got away with that attempt, pulled a string of robberies, and were finally caught in a police stakeout.

After doing his time and being released, Bill largely stayed clean and, after two years, I helped him get off parole.

About a year after that, Bill's mother called me late one night, very distraught. "Bill's using drugs again," she said.

"He's mentioned you often and trusts you. Would you try to see him, talk to him, get him to stop?" I called the number she gave me. A woman answered. I gave my name and said I'd like to talk to Bill. The woman said she was Bill's wife, that Bill wasn't there, but she'd give him the message. Bill dropped by my office the next morning. I hardly recognized him, his appearance was so changed. He seemed greatly amused at my reaction to his new "straight" image, but said he had responsibilities now and had had to clean up his act. He then asked me why I'd called. I told him of his mother's call and concern, and asked him if there was anything to it. He said that he had not been involved with drugs of any kind, but that his mother suffered an obsessional fear he would go back on dope. I told him that his mother had been worried to the point of incoherence and suggested that he talk to her. He did so. As it turned out, her misplaced concern over Bill combined with a host of other problems had pushed her to the point where she snapped, and was hospitalized briefly for psychiatric treatment. She was able to return to work after a short period of therapy. In both Bill's and Elena's cases, the problem existed with the parent. Elena does not recognize or acknowledge her difficulty, and until she does nothing much will happen. She may never face up to the fact that she is an alcoholic because her pattern of withdrawing and avoiding contact will probably not result in externally caused crises or trouble. Elena's mother sees the situation for what it is and wants to do something to promote or provoke change in Elena, but has so far failed.

Bill's behavior at an earlier time had left his mother with a problem that she had still not resolved. It persisted in her imagination, although Bill seems to have succeeded in shedding his old habits. But his mother, threatened by her recollections and greatly troubled by difficulties at work and at home, invented the reason for calling me, perhaps to draw attention to her own plight. Her anxiety was real and severe, but baseless.

Origins

The reasons for the excessive use of drugs are manifold. The effects may either reduce or eliminate a malign state— depression, anomie, irritability, vulnerability—in the individual or induce a pleasant one—optimism, euphoria, feelings of power, potency, authority. Just those effects alone would be enough for many individuals to develop drug dependencies of one kind or another.

Though there is nothing especially new about drug abuse, the extent to which it has permeated American life in recent times is significant and frightening. As the pace of change accelerates, as the dance of life becomes faster and more intricate, as the ability of the individual to control and regulate his or her own affairs erodes, drugs seem to offer the user powerful alternative realities. The hectic pace of life, the alienation, the sense of loss of control encourages the increased use of all kinds of substances to produce by turns serenity, high energy, dreamlike peace, or a sense of personal command. Technological change has made much of this possible with the discovery of an assortment of new mood-influencing substances. These chemicals, first introduced to manage psychiatric disorders, have lately brought about an enormous reduction in the numbers of individuals confined to mental hospitals. When administered in smaller dosages they control less severe or disabling complaints, lifting depressions or reducing anxiety reactions, making it possible for individuals suffering what had once been disabling psychological conditions to return to the community at large. Significant numbers of people began to use them and "uppers" and "downers" soon found their way into the illicit drug trade.

Development and widespread use of these mood-altering prescription drugs owes much to the belief that pervades medicine, and indeed all of society, that taking doses of a "healing" substance is the best or most appropriate means of controlling or managing symptoms. Though this approach often produces valuable social and economic results, one consequence has been an increasing degree of drug dependency; another has been to foster the idea that the solution to most human problems may be found in a bottle or syringe.

Accompanying the medical developments was the dramatic evolution of a youth culture in which drugs play a significant social role. Here the emphasis has been more on experiencing states that were mind- or consciousness-expanding, that remove the constraints imposed by the existing culture. LSD, whose effects were first studied because it produced symptoms similar to those encountered in schizophrenia, found its way onto the streets.

Marijuana and hashish, which had been known for millenia, came into common use, and other more insidious drugs, such as heroin, cocaine, the amphetamines, or PCP, also began to enjoy wide circulation.

Alcohol also achieves some of the inhibition-freeing, mood-loosening influences of the psychotropic chemicals, and its use has grown steadily over the years. The proportion of individuals who drink alcohol has grown by nearly 25% in the past 40 years; the per capita consumption of alcohol has quadrupled in that time.

Drugs and alcohol provide a superior sense of ease and comfort. They free individuals from the present, or permit them the illusion of controlling it. They also represent the largest and most costly social problem on the American scene. Interestingly, a drug, Soma, appeared on pharmacy shelves not too long ago. The substance used in Huxley's *Brave New World* to induce states of satisfaction and well-being in the population, and thus to enable the leaders to maintain control, was also called "soma."

Getting Help

Getting help for individuals abusing acohol or drugs—or for those affected by those individuals—is particularly difficult. You, the parent, are faced, first, with the need to be sure that the child is abusing the substance, whatever it may be. Often the user is not aware of his or her dependency or is able, honestly if wrongly, to deny the existence of a problem. The individual who each day consumes a couple of sixpacks of beer will contend that since only beer is consumed and since beer does not contain a great deal of alcohol, there is no problem of heavy drinking. Deception also plays a part. Drinkers often understate the amount of alcohol they consume, deluding themselves and others. Observers impose their own standards of judgment, adding yet another complication. For some, any consumption of alcohol at all represents excessive use.

For help in defining alcohol abuse, inquire at the local office of the nationwide network of Alcoholism Councils to elicit information that should help decide precisely when and whether a problem may be said to exist and, if so, what to do about it. This and other alcohol treatment facilities are generally listed under "Alcohol" in the yellow pages of your telephone directory.

In addition, many employers have become aware of the economic costs of alcoholism and have established treatment programs for their employees. These have proved to be among the more successful responses to the problem, and should always be considered as possible solutions. The Alcohol Council will know which employers in their area offer such programs.

Other individuals victimized by drug or alcohol abuse by a member of the family—the abuser's spouse or children in particular—have often found AL-ANON (for adults) helpful in providing comfort, understanding, and knowledge of how to help themselves and, indirectly, their alcoholic relatives. ALATEEN strives to accomplish the same goals for teenage children caught up in a family situation with one or more alcoholic members. AL-ANON and ALATEEN are listed in the white pages of the phone book.

If there is real physical danger to the substance abuser's small children, danger that originates with carelessness or neglect on the part of substance-abusing parents, the children should be taken away from the parents for their own safety and well-being. A conference with representatives of the Alcoholism Council, juvenile authorities, or other legal counsel will reveal the steps and procedures necessary to accomplish this.

When excessive use of drugs is involved and if prescription drugs are being abused, the physician responsible for the dosage should be contacted directly. The doctor should be talked to in person. In approaching the physician, the parent should be prepared to state the amount of use, the symptoms, and the reason for concern.

When over-the-counter or street drugs are involved, most communities support free clinics, drug treatment centers, or drug diversion programs. These are listed under "Drugs" in the yellow pages. State Departments of Health maintain directories of drug referral, emergency treatment, or rehabilitation services. A phone call or letter should tell you what is available in your area. Free clinics are especially likely to be knowledgeable and forthright in offering suggestions and advice.

When street drugs are concerned, one common difficulty is found in the conflicting attitudes that parents and children have about the use of substances like marijuana. Parents are likely to have intense fears about the effects of "pot," condemning it out of all proportion to its dangers. The use of any drug is cause for alarm, but Dr. Benjamin Spock has said that marijuana is much, much less harmful than heroin, the amphetamines, the barbiturates, LSD, alcohol, and tobacco.

Getting control over substances that create either physical or psychological dependency is extremely difficult and some authorities (AA for example) do not use the word "cure" in describing the outcomes of treatment. Little is known about the mechanisms of dependency.

You can probably best help in resolving the problem by pulling back from it. Authorities have long known that individuals who do use alcohol or drugs to excess are often unknowingly supported or nurtured in their habits by those close to them. AA calls these people "enablers." Elena's mother, by paying the rent, makes it easier for Elena to hold on to her alcoholism. Realization that one is part of an unintended conspiracy comes hard; taking the resolute action necessary to break it up is even harder. Nevertheless, forcing the child to face up to and take full responsibility for its actions is ultimately a caring, loving act. Tolerating, covering up for, or denying someone's dependency or addiction will only prolong it.

Help in taking the difficult step of detaching yourself from your substance-abusing child can be secured from individual or group counseling sources or from the AL-ANON groups already mentioned. Although they will not get rid of the problem, they can provide insight into it. They can also do much to clarify your relationship to what is indisputably the child's problem, helping you to handle anxiety and self-blame more comfortably, and allowing for a more detached, dispassionate view of the matter.

CHAPTER 17

THE UNGRATEFUL CHILD

> *How sharper than a serpent's tooth it is*
> *To have a thankless child!*

Introduction

What children do often troubles their parents; what they do not do frequently troubles them more. Neglecting parents is one of these hurtful acts of omission.

"Honor thy father and thy mother..." the commandment goes, and parents do come to expect that their middle and later years will be lived out serenely and with due respect and attention from their children. When the expectation fails—when contacts between parents and children are few, brief, and perfunctory—the parents are likely to feel hurt and cheated.

Wanda, widowed, is in her early sixties. Her two children, both married, live at a considerable distance. They rarely write or call, and almost never visit. When Wanda asks why they do not come to see her, they reply that they have trouble getting away (both partners in both couples work) and that the trip would be too long and too expensive.

Wanda has become more and more depressed and upset, constantly dwelling on the scant contact she has had with her children and grandchildren. In talking with her, I learned that she lives alone in a small apartment, does not work, has no hobbies, no church affiliation, and few friends. She does not meet people easily. She spends most of her time watching television. Lately she has been going to bed very early and sleeping for long periods, often thirteen or fourteen hours per night.

Her behavior was petulant and critical throughout our first interviews. She did little but whine and complain about her children and the way they were treating her after all she had done for them. "That's the thanks I get," she said, over and over.

I began to understand why the children had been remiss about keeping in close touch with Wanda. Even for only fifty minutes a week she was hard to take.

Without going into the details of how the change was brought about—the process involved weekly incremental assignments in making overtures to other people and in changing her habitual patterns—she began to develop some skill and confidence in meeting people and to develop a more active social life. At the same time she came to the important realization that contact with her children was a two-way street and that if she wanted to see them she could go where they were. Better so, since she had the time and the means to live comfortably and to travel if she wished. By now she had the fortitude to approach the children directly to say that she would like to come on a visit and to ask when and for how long it would be convenient.

The trip had some rough patches, but it turned out very well on the whole. The children were surprised and pleased at the changes they saw in Wanda and, following the visit, they apparently felt more motivated to keep in touch. For Wanda's part, with her life becoming more involved and busy she caught herself thinking that it wasn't too late for another try at the brass ring. And doing so, she lost much of her preoccupation with the children, and why they were ignoring her. Of late, they probably hear no more out of her than she does from them.

Origins

Not seeing or hearing from adult children often enough is a common complaint made by middle-aged parents. It is also one of the more painful ones.

The ties between adult children and their parents are not so close as they once might have been because of several social factors we have already touched on—breakup of the extended family, increased mobility of the population, evolution of a youth culture that has weakened the intergenerational links, and the availability of improved, more varied social programs that help the older generation to maintain their fiscal and physical independence. Both the possibility and the need for intimate daily contact between the generations have declined.

In addition, the mode of keeping in touch has changed. The middle-aged parent is much more likely to rely on letters; the child uses the telephone. Even if the child telephones with some regularity, the empty-handed return trips from the mail box add up to the conclusion that one is being neglected.

Honoring parents makes a good deal of sense in static, authoritarian societies; in dynamic, professedly egalitarian, youth-oriented ones like the United States it does not. Yet the parents have been nurtured on a commandment that harks back to an earlier, different time. As they see it, it is their right to have the child's attention—and it is the responsibility of the child to give it—a give and take arrangement, with the parent getting and the child giving. The child, nurtured under different circumstances doesn't see matters in quite the same way.

After all, he or she has problems and responsibilities, demands on time and energy, with none of the advantages that life in an extended family conferred—shared responsibility for the care of the children, cooperation and collaboration in carrying out household chores, and the like.

This does not mean that everything was rosy in days gone by. One of my own vivid childhood memories is my grandmother's routine question when I returned from the daily trip to the post office: "Anything for me?"

Almost always I would have to answer "No." Her disappointment never failed to show. She was ever hoping for a letter from my uncle, her only surviving son and her favorite child. He wrote perhaps four times a year and even though the old woman lived in a home with her daughter, her son-in-law, and her grandchildren, the sense of being neglected and unwanted was powerful and painful for her.

Being ignored is not the inevitable lot of today's middle-aged parent, but the ghettoization and compartmentalization of the generations is a strong social trend that often produces individual feelings of isolation and abandonment, of disappointment and anger at the ungrateful child.

Dealing With Feelings of Neglect

Remedies do exist. One important alternative is to take advantage of the many opportunities to declare one's own independence and to refashion for yourself a life that does not center on unrealistic and unfair demands and expectations of the children.

Social, recreational, and educational opportunities are proliferating, and in many places there is an extraordinary variety of programs available for the asking. Many educational institutions, faced with declining enrollments in their traditional programs, are tailoring courses and curricula with the interests and needs of the young-old or the old-old in mind.

Voluntary organizations, religious groups, and local governments also provide facilities and devise programs sufficiently diverse that the older person has the opportunity to select from and participate in a rich variety of activities. These offer fellowship, recreational activity, training in social skills, handicrafts, cultural activities, travel, and the like.

Organizations that speak to the problems and needs of seniors and capitalize on their skills and experience exist everywhere. They range from the political and social activism of the Gray Panthers to the nationwide network of senior volunteer programs. There are almost limitless alternatives to moping around waiting for that occasional letter or phone call from an adult child.

It is also possible to do something more than bury one's hurt beneath an avalanche of frantic activity. Admitting that the expectations we hold for our adult children may be out of touch with the times, and recognizing that it is unrealistic to place responsibility for taking initiative entirely on the child, the parent is freed to act directly. Wanda proved to have enough gumption to take matters into her own hands with what proved to be satisfying results.

In initiating direct action, you should have a clear and fair understanding of conditions as they are now, how you would like to see them changed, and what you are able and willing to do to help bring about the changes. Making unilateral demands from an authoritarian or "owed to me" position is not likely to bring about much real reform although it may force a grudging and even mean-spirited compliance.

Apart from fashioning a new lifestyle that deemphasizes dependence on one's children, or redefines the nature, direction, and responsibility for maintaining and nourishing the relationship, the parent can work to achieve the wise, loving tolerance that Erikson identifies as the full fruition of the earlier stages of development. Understanding that children act out of causes or reasons that do not signify rejection or lack of care or concern for their parents is an important aspect of maturity. Love and understanding are the most important gifts a parent can bring to a child, regardless of the time of life.

PART FIVE

Coping Strategies

This last section of *Coping with Your Grown Children* presents a rational model to follow in dealing with family conflicts. The model requires the same degree of study and attention that a rudimentary repair or instruction manual might demand. I believe that with this minimal effort you will readily be able to grasp—and put into practice—the principles and procedures presented here. To help you understand and apply the process, each stage is carefully defined, described, and illustrated in Chapter 18. Following this detailed exposition, Chapter 19 takes you though a step-by-step exercise in which you apply the method directly to your own situation.

The model assumes that parents and children are, or may be, able and willing to approach their differences openly and thoughtfully, treating each other's individual rights with respect, and holding the welfare of all those involved as a primary consideration. The greatest obstacles to rational resolution of parent–child conflict are the intense feelings associated with the problem and the entangled relationships of the parties.

The emotions set loose by parent–grown child problems all too often provoke rash, ill-considered, and destructive reactions. The decision-making process I have outlined here offers a structured alternative to this type of impulsive, off-hand maneuver. A serious, determined effort to apply such rational methods to the resolution of your interpersonal conflicts will yield you many more affirmative outcomes than shoot-from-the-hip efforts ever will.

Throughout, we have stressed the importance of admitting the need for and the desirability of seeking outside help.

The final Chapter 20 will show you how to decide whether you need such help in the first place, and will then outline procedures to follow in locating and selecting the right kind of aid. It also contains a comprehensive annotated list of key helping resources likely to be found in nearly every community.

Taking the time to figure out precisely what type of assistance one needs, and what kinds are actually available, will increase the likelihood that help—whatever form it finally takes—will be effective. Suffering problems is part of everyone's life. Enduring them because of the stubborn belief that one is somehow a better person for going it alone is silly to the point of self-destructiveness.

CHAPTER 18

HOW TO DEVELOP A RATIONAL SOLUTION FOR YOUR PARENT–CHILD PROBLEM
Building a Decision Tree

> *He who will not reason is a bigot:*
> *he who cannot is a fool;*
> *and he who dares not is a slave.*

Introduction

You can make better, more informed decisions about problems with your adult children—and most other problems in life, for that matter—if you pay attention to a very few fundamental principles of decision-making. Those principles—and a procedure that will help you observe them—is what this chapter is all about. The process sketched here calls for the construction of a decision tree, which is a problem-handling method that has been widely applied in business or administrative decision-making processes. What first attracted me to it was the ready correspondence of the method with the way the best psychologists and others were solving human dilemmas. But before getting down to the details, let me sketch the most important points to keep in mind. They are three.

1. Family problems are complex. They involve several different individuals, each of whom views a problem situation from his or her own unique standpoint. Thus, the participants may not agree on anything beyond admitting that something is indeed wrong. A few may go so far as to deny that anything at all is the matter. And worse still, the problem may itself be imaginary, existing only in the fear-filled, disordered imagination of one of the parties.

2. Conflict is inherent in family disputes. Because interpersonal conflict is central to the dispute, there is always the danger of acting impulsively, irrationally, or without consulting others, simply to escape one's feelings of distress.

3. Sometimes a solution does not work out. Even with the most careful analysis, it may prove impossible to anticipate either the reactions of other individuals or the ongoing unpredictabilities that crop up in any given situation. Thus what appears on first viewing to be the best, most workable solution to a problem may well misfire. If that happens, it is imperative to remember that your planned remedy was the best that could be devised at the time and with the information then available. Given the unforeseen nature of the later events, it is unlikely that any other approach would have been more effective.

By remembering that problems between middle-aged parents and adult children are complex, emotionally charged, and (sometimes) irresolvable, frustration and anger can be avoided or kept within tolerable limits on all sides.

Principles of Decision-Making

When it comes to finding the way out of a thicket of difficulties with your adult children, heeding the following list of "Rules" will ease matters. There are five such principles:

1. Open up the lines of communication. This is, by far, the most important principle. It commands you to speak out honestly and openly about the difficulty—as you see it and as it affects you—and equally binds you to listen *attentively* to the others involved. Communicating in this open manner is an essential prerequisite to constructive resolution of your parent–grown child conflicts, much as it is in every area of human intercourse.

Achieving open, matter-of-fact communication is essential, though extremely difficult to accomplish, given our individual differences in perceptions, temperaments, and tempers. Communication here means clarifying and (when appropriate) conveying information about your own thoughts and feelings, as well as learning everything you can about the thoughts and feelings of the others involved in the situation that is troubling you. Communicating is not blaming or censuring. It does not occur when you indulge in the useless luxury, however satisfying, of telling the other person off, either face-to-face or in your fantasies. It is a process that has as its goal greater understanding and appreciation of the several viewpoints involved. If the individuals caught up in a family problem are unable to abide by this principle—if open statements and civil discussion largely free from criticism, ordering, or bullying are not possible—then there is little prospect of resolving the matter. It will either persist or it will be replaced by something worse, as in the following case:

> Matt got involved in a sexual escapade that resulted in a criminal charge being filed against him. His parents engaged a lawyer, but the father, a stern, punitive, and unforgiving man, condemned Matt in excessively harsh and brutal terms. Matt committed suicide just before his case came to trial. The mother blames the father for Matt's suicide and the father is now wracked with guilt.

The need for communication is present whether the underlying parent–grown child problem is shared or individual. For problems shared among parents and children, this need should be self-evident, but such openness is no less important when the parents alone find themselves troubled. It is essential to try to understand one's own problem. Giving it voice, talking it out, helps in the preliminary process of clarification and resolution. Talking a problem out may also alert others to your needs, and thereby bring about changes in external circumstances that will contribute to the resolution of at least some elements of the problem.

Mr. and Ms. Abbott only saw their oldest son, Gary, on special occasions. This bothered them a great deal and they decided to discuss their feelings with Gary and his wife, Peggy. The discussion brought out the fact that Gary and Peggy were striving to divide their time fairly between both sets of parents. They also had many other demands on their free time, demands of which Mr. and Ms. Abbott were quite unaware. Gary and Peggy, for their part, felt extremely pressured and guilty about the way things were going. As a result of the frank exchange of ideas, the two couples were able to arrange to come together under more flexible and satisfying conditions.

2. *Act on problems before they get of hand.* Turning away from a conflict in the hope that it will vanish sometimes—but quite rarely—pays off. It is a tactic that only encourages problems to grow ever more prickly and unmanageable.

When a grown child–parent problem first becomes evident, then is the time to do something about it. It may turn out to be only temporary and trivial—soon to evaporate. Fine. By acting immediately, you will have discovered the solution all the more quickly than you might have if you had only waited and temporized. And if the difficulty proves not to be a small matter, then you are working on a solution at a time when conditions are much more malleable than they will later become.

3. *Address the conflict rationally.* Interpersonal conflicts are best dealt with in an orderly, systematic way—one that

aims at making the soundest decision possible. Setting in motion a rational process designed to understand and solve a parent–grown child problem is likely to be more constructive over the long haul than one focused on satisfying such understandable but counterproductive personal goals as getting even or having one's own way. Though there is a bitter satisfaction in being able to say "I told you so!", avoiding the temptation to do so will keep everyone's attention centered on the problem and thus is far more likely to lead to productive solutions.

4. Use advice. The ties between parents and children are based on long and close familiarity. Long acquaintanceship means that one gets to to know other persons' habits intimately, and encourages the belief that it is possible to forecast how that person will behave, at any place or time. Such confidence is unwarranted for most members of our wayward species, as well as excessively limiting—people can, and therefore are likely to, spring surprises. Because of the nature of the parent–child relationship, you as parent may not always be fully capable of dealing with your child and the problem he or she represents in a sensitive, rational way. Accordingly, obtaining a second opinion from an independent, neutral person may well help clarify your problem with your child, and point to possible solutions. Such a consultant/confidant can be anyone who is trustworthy, just so long as it is not one who will unquestioningly swallow your viewpoint. You need an umpire, a mediator, not an echo.

5. Get help when it's needed. When communication between parents and their grown children seems impossible or extremely difficult, when action seems stalled, when you cannot proceed rationally, or when friends tell you that you are not acting sensibly, it is certainly time to seek professional help. The final chapter describes the kinds of help available for particular types of parent–child conflicts and outlines how to go about securing the best kind of assistance available.

Solving Problems Rationally

We wish now to present a rational method for dealing with interpersonal conflict. It uses a "decision tree," which is nothing more than an orderly, step-by-step procedure to follow in arriving at a solution. You will see that it actually entails making a series of choices. To arrive at a place where you can take a major resolving step, it is usually necessary to begin with one or a series of smaller moves. You should bear in mind that no two trees—and certainly no two decision trees —are exactly alike. The decision path that one finally follows will always be determined by the specific elements of the situation—the people involved, the severity and duration of the problem, the intensity of the feelings, and so on.

Decision-tree solutions are "optimal"; that is, when carefully constructed and acted upon, they seek to produce the best possible outcome. The process presented below also permits the decision-maker to do the next best thing by equipping him or her to select a "good enough" alternative from among all of those that might be possible. This type of solution has been called a "satisficer"; it is adequate (it satisfies), but not perfect. Though determining what might constitute a good enough solution is not as desirable as finding the best, that "best" solution may be out of the question because the problem is either too severe or too complicated to permit implementation of an ideal solution.

The steps in a rational decision-making or conflict-resolving process are described below and in Figure 3:

1. Define the problem
2. Identify the 'ideal solution'
3. Decide whether the 'ideal solution' is feasible
4. If the 'ideal solution' is not possible, identify acceptable 'alternative solutions'
5. Formulate methods or strategies to achieve the 'ideal' (or 'alternative') solutions
6. Determine the 'anticipated consequence' (positive and negative) for each solution

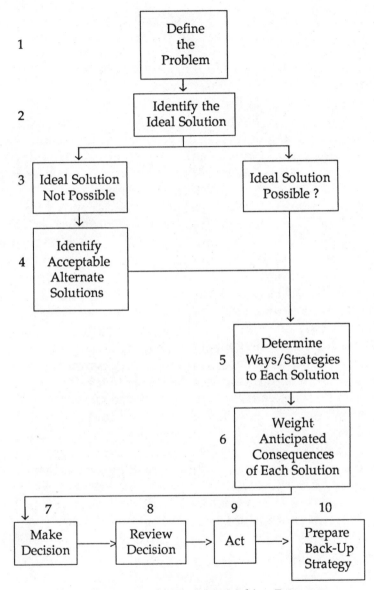

Fig. 3. Steps in the Decision-Making Process

7. Make a tentative decision
8. Review (with consultation) all steps leading to the decision
9. Act
10. Have a back-up strategy available in case the first solution fails

To illustrate how this process works, we will now apply it, step-by step, to the following situation.

Your healthy 23-year-old son, Al, is still not out on his own. He continues to live at home and gives no signs at all of wanting to move on. He has completed his education, and he is physically, intellectually, and emotionally sound. Al is an ingratiating and likable guy and you and your spouse are both extremely fond of him, a feeling he reciprocates. He works 20 hours per week as a sales clerk in a record store, but what he earns there is not enough to support him on his own. He is not looking seriously for a full-time job and he does not contribute to the household upkeep. You get by comfortably, although the money has to be watched carefully. You are concerned, both because Al is seemingly not taking responsibility for himself and, in addition, because you are beginning to be preoccupied with your own mid-life plans, with the idea of doing some traveling, and with providing for your retirement years. There is only one other child at home now, Rick, a senior in high school. You and your spouse have talked the matter over carefully, and have agreed that—for his own good and for yours too—it would be better if Al were to take charge of his own life. In the course of reaching this conclusion you have used the procedures of fantasizing and projecting that were spelled out in Chapter 4. From them, you have concluded that you should do something before the problem gets worse—or before you start making it into something worse than it already is. Your feelings are best described as those of upset and concern. You are not angry with Al; merely impatient with him because he doesn't have his act together. Neither you nor your spouse has talked directly or openly with Al about the situation.

Step 1: *Defining the Problem*

From your standpoint the problem is clear; you think that it is time that Al became responsible for himself. By not being out on his own you believe that he is hurting himself and that he is also beginning to complicate and interfere with your own hopes and plans for the future. You believe, further, that you have discharged your responsibilities to him, having seen to his education, and having provided the material and psychological support he needed as he was growing up.

Step 2: Identifying the 'Ideal Solution'

The 'ideal solution' is equally obvious: Al moves out, establishing his own economic and personal independence with as little damage to family feelings and relationships as possible.

Step 3: Deciding Whether the Ideal Solution Is Feasible

Since most children do eventually leave home and make it on their own, and since there is nothing obviously wrong with Al, you conclude that nothing stands in the way of the ideal solution. You now know what you wish to do; the problem lies only in deciding precisely how you want to get there.

However, you also recognize that your version of the ideal solution is one-sided. You know that there may be matters you are quite unaware of that will interfere with implementing the ideal solution. To be on the safe side, you visualize some alternative solutions that might be tolerable from your standpoint.

Step 4: Identifying Acceptable Alternative Solutions

First, think of as many possibilities as you can. Here are some of the options and the way you might analyze each one.

Alternative	Advantages	Disadvantages
1. Do nothing*	Al won't be upset	The problem will persist and you'll feel worse
2. Let Al continue to stay at home under a revised set of rules	Eases your financial and work load	Doesn't really put Al in charge of himself

(continued)

Alternative	Advantages	Disadvantages
	May motivate Al to get out on his own	Equitable rules are hard to work out and even harder to stick with
3. Help Al to set up on his own (with or without an ending date)	Al moves to the place where he must be marginally more self-sufficient	This gets rid of Al by throwing money at him. It may actually compound the difficulty by creating a different kind of dependency. It could make aspects of your problem worse
4. Get outside help for Al	Brings in an experienced person May get Al going	Al may not need outside help Al may not want the help and may be unwilling to accept it Help costs money Help doesn't always work
5. Get outside help for yourselves	Makes you feel better	Doesn't help Al with his problem *Still costs money*
6. Get outside help for yourselves and Al	See 4 & 5 above	See 4 & 5 above

*Doing nothing is always an alternative and, if selected, is the one most likely to prove harmful in the long run. If a problem is recognized to exist, it should be addressed. Otherwise it will drag on and probably get worse.

None of these alternatives is especially attractive, but second best is often unappealing.

Step 5: Formulating Strategies to Achieve the Ideal Solution

There are a number of different routes by which Al may be gotten out on his own. These can be thought of as either immediate or deferred solutions, as well as ones that are arrived at through either unilateral action (by you acting alone without consultation with Al) or via bilateral action with Al's direct involvement. At this stage it is vital to try to imagine as many different paths to the Ideal Solution as possible. Even so, you may not be able to discern every alternative, but careful consideration at this stage and the next one will help to avoid rash and destructive actions.

In Al's case, the options are listed in the brief table below:

Type of action	Immediate	Deferred
Unilateral	Kick him out	Serve notice that he will have to get out (with or without a deadline)
Bilateral	Agreement to leave now (with or without conditions or commitments from either side)	Agreement to leave at some future time (contingent on achieving conditions making the departure possible)

Note well that getting to the ideal solution may require passing through several intervening steps. Disposing of a complex problem is not like tossing out yesterday's newspaper. Agreement that Al will leave when (as soon as) he finds work that will support him entails a substrategy, which is "finding work." And, to find work, several additional steps may be required, each calling for some sort of decision or action on the part of the parents.

By this time, the analysis has progressed to the point at which it is possible to begin sketching a "decision tree." This has been done in Figure 4. It represents the problem and the steps taken so far to resolve it.

Step 6: Determining Anticipated Consequences

Each stratagem that you have identified in the preceding section will have both positive and negative consequences.

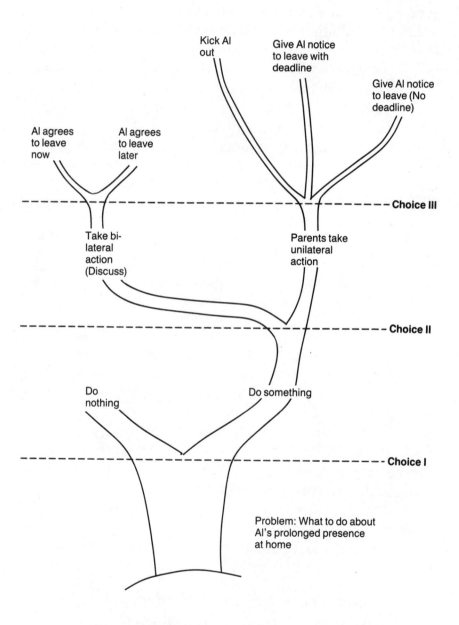

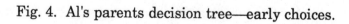

Fig. 4. Al's parents decision tree—early choices.

The one you finally elect to follow will be that which promises the best balance of favorable and unfavorable outcomes.

In Al's case the analysis of consequences might look like this:

Stratagem	Pluses	Minuses
Kick him out	Gets Al on his own right now	Arbitrary
		Likely to damage the good relationship between you. Doesn't deal with Al's problem, whatever it is.
		May actually be harmful to Al
Give him a firm deadline to get out	Promises a definite end to *your* problem	Arbitrary
		May damage the good relationship between you
		If Al doesn't move by the deadline you will be forced either to kick him out or to extend the deadline
		Doesn't deal with Al's problem—simply tells him he has one and has X time to do something about it
		By placing additional stress on Al, may actually intensify the difficulty
Agreement to leave now	Gets Al out	Since Al is not self-supporting, you may have to help
	Since the decision is mutual, risk of bad feeling is reduced	Doesn't deal with Al's problem
		May damage the existing relationship
Agreement to leave at some future time	Gives a definite but agreed-on deadline	Stretches things out
		May require time, money and help from you
	Addresses itself to Al's problem constructively	
	Is least likely to harm the relationship with Al	

Consideration of the consequences permits expansion of the decision tree; this has been done in Figure 5.

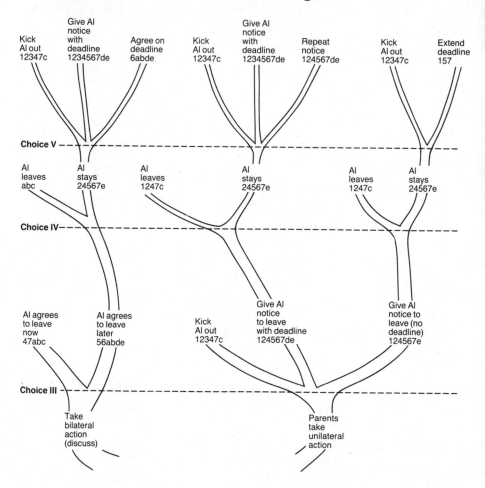

Fig. 5. Al's parents' decision tree—later choices and their consequences. *Negative features*: 1. Arbitrary; 2. Risks causing bad feelings; 3. Ignores Al's problem; 4. May harm Al; 5. Delays action and resolution; 6. May require help from you; 7. May harm you. *Positive features*: a. Consensual (mutually agreed-on); b. Holds risk of bad feelings to a minimum; c. Gets Al out on his own at the time action occurs; d. Establishes definite time to act; e. Gives opportunity for constructive action.

In this circumstance it seems clear that the most promising and least harmful alternative would be to work toward a bilateral, deferred solution. In this eventuality, the parents would want to sit down with Al and express their feelings openly and without rancor. After all, they aren't feeling angry about the issue and should be able to talk to Al without losing control. This should permit them to unearth any aspects of the problem that they don't now know about and to encourage Al to obtain the right kind of assistance. Al's problem may be that:

1. He just never thought about getting out on his own. He likes being at home *or*
2. He has thought about it and has tried unsuccessfully to find work. He knows what he wants to do and where he wants to go *or*
3. He has thought about it and has tried to find work and has been disappointed in his search. He is not sure of what he wants to do or how to go about finding out *or*
4. He is afraid of being turned down or of failing *or*
5. He has no idea about how, when, or where to start

Each of these problems should be approached differently. It is obvious that outside help is likely to be needed with any of them if Al is to become physically and economically independent of home and parents. This may take time, but even the knowledge that the issue is out in the open, that Al is aware of how if affects you and is doing something about it, may help the situation look—and feel—much better.

The analysis of these circumstances—of the problem, the strategies, the solutions, and the consequences—will be determined predominantly by the individuals involved and the kinds of relationships they have. The Al in our example is one problem; another Al in another situation with another set of parents might be an entirely different matter. If Al were a surly, lazy, insolent troublemaker, if his parents were having serious financial problems, both the analysis and the conclusions would necessarily be different. Under those circumstances, kicking Al out right now might be the best solution.

Step 7: *Making a Tentative Decision*

Having figured out the nature of the problem, the desired solution, the strategies available, and the consequences of each stratagem, you are now in a position to decide what to do. The decision ought to favor the alternative that has the most favorable balance of positive (in relation to negative) consequences. In Al's case, the best approach is the bilateral decision involving discussion leading to an agreement on his part to leave when certain intermediate goals are attained. As a general (but by no means universal) rule, solutions arrived at jointly after full and open discussion are much more likely to be free of the destructive consequences that often attend conflict between adult children and their parents.

Step 8: *Reviewing the Decision*

For several reasons—the complexity of the problems and the interrelationships of the individuals involved; or possibly the difficulty of thinking about or weighing the consequences of the various strategies before putting the decision to work— you need to take time carefully to review what you have done. At this point it may be prudent to submit the analysis to a friend or confidant in order to hear an independent opinion about what has been done. Is your definition of the problem fair? What about the solutions? Are they feasible? Are there others you have overlooked? Are your strategies sound? Have you thought of all the consequences? Is your decision the best or most promising one?

In seeking consultation, keep in mind that this process too can be carried to excess. Some troubled individuals compulsively seek advice from a variety of sources and, when conflicting suggestions emerge, wind up more confused and unsure of themselves than when they began. Others want only to have their conclusions confirmed and continue looking for someone who will give them a vote of confidence. Knowing of these pitfalls will help you avoid them. Limit your appeals for help to an individual or individuals who you are confident can give you an informed opinion—and once they have delivered it, make a point of considering it most carefully. Ministers or other religious figures will often prove helpful, since they will have had experience and training in dealing with similar problems. A relative—even another child—may be able to point to flaws or omissions in what you have done.

Step 9: Taking Action

Once you have made and reviewed your decision, act! Nothing will be gained by waiting. Unless you do something, the problem will persist and, because you are now much more aware of it, only grow worse.

And once you act, adhere to your plan of action unless something happens to convince you beyond any doubt that your decision was catastrophically wrong. Nothing that you do will confuse an issue more than declaring a course of action, and then backing away from it. Vacillation will not only complicate matters; it will also make any future action all the more difficult.

In Al's case, a conference that establishes the steps to be taken and defines the obligations of everyone concerned would be a worthwhile first step. The conference should result in an agreement (perhaps subject to later renegotiation, depending on how things went) that will chart out the strategies by which Al will become self-sufficient. These steps might include vocational counseling and career planning, help in locating and securing appropriate work, assistance in overcoming some of the difficulties he will inevitably encounter in getting down to the task of becoming independent, working out financial and other details of the move-out, and the like. Finally, you would concur on a time by which the process would be completed and add any other codicils that might be required. If the process is going to take money, for example, who is to put it up? If Al is to bear the cost, but cannot come up with the money now, how will he repay you? And so on. Try to cover all the eventualities, the intervening steps to the ideal solution, and have a clear understanding about them, what they are to be, when, how, under what auspices they will take place, and whose responsibility they are.

Finally, with a course of action lined out, try to develop a constructive, supportive posture. It is easy to become pushy, continually worrying at the problem, nagging. Providing for periodic reports of progress through discussion is the best antidote to this tendency. Since there are likely to be disappointments and setbacks, strive to be encouraging, supportive, and positive. Even if Al does not succeed in his first job interview, he will learn something from it and it is possible to put aside the disappointment to identify and examine the positive things that did transpire.

Step 10: Developing a Backup Stratagem

Even the best-laid plans sometimes go wrong and you may then find yourself the disappointed owner of a solution that failed to work. Admitting that possibility and allowing for it beforehand will help considerably in managing your own frustration if failure does happen and it also provides a potentially viable substitute plan.

Here you will probably find that one of the alternatives you considered earlier would be an acceptable second best solution. It is also possible that, in working toward the preferred solution, you will uncover serious unanticipated problems that force changes in your strategies and deadlines.

Having an idea about how you will handle Al's failure to find work will make it easier to deal with if it actually happens. Acknowledging and taking into account the unlikely prospect that Al might be unable to live up to his end of the agreement will permit you to formulate some definite courses of action in advance of the event.

It is possible for a parent not to involve the child in working out an action plan. Such unilateral solutions will probably work only poorly if they do not fail altogether. Though the process, as we have presented it, permits such an approach, open discussion with all of those concerned can occur at any stage. If something does not seem quite right, this concern can be put forth for discussion without having a definite idea about what is wrong or knowing what, if anything, can be done about it.

When the situation is such that airing or introducing these questions is not possible—because, for instance, the home environment does not allow such concerns to be raised —then the home situation itself needs work. And because it has been a long time in developing, it may in fact prove next to impossible to change it. Asking an authoritarian, impatient, irascible, dogmatic father who expects to be obeyed instantly and without question to participate productively in an open discussion is unrealistic. Expecting a defiant, rebellious son— one who has always acted as if the experiences of others have no validity for him—to discuss his (and your) problem openly and freely is equally unrealistic.

In short, personal or situational factors may at times all but rule out the possibility of fruitful discussions leading to shared or consensual solutions. When such conditions prevail, the problem will often simply remain unresolved and troubling, or possibly force unilateral action with consequent damage to interpersonal relationships. When the problem does persist, or is replaced by an equally painful situation, the troubled individuals are left alone to manage their own feelings and reactions. *If you can't solve the problem, it is essential to work at changing the way you feel about it.* (See Chapter 3.)

Another Example

Al's case provides a relatively easy, conflict-free illustration of the decision-tree method. As it turned out, the real-life Al simply enjoyed being at home. He was having a good, easy-going time and he just was not ready to settle down. When he realized that he was giving his parents concern, as well as upsetting their own hopes and plans, he was extremely contrite and immediately began looking for work. Finding suitable employment proved to be much more difficult than he had expected it to be, but his parents gave him a good deal of help and support. He finally landed a job that, though not exactly what he had expected or hoped for, did permit him to strike out on his own. It took him six months and he and his parents experienced some ups and downs before things finally worked out.

Presented below is another, more complex, situation, one that actually consists of a collection of individual problems with different and (in some instances) incompatible 'ideal solutions.' Here the discussion has been kept to a minimum in order to present a clearer picture of the step-like evolution of the decision-making process.

Step 1: The Situation

Susan, the older child and only daughter of Ted and Vi, has disclosed that she is living with Ty. Susan, 24, lives in a town 50 miles from the parental home and works full-time as a nurse. The man she is living with is a Japanese-American. He is 26 and has his own prospering photographic business. Neither Susan nor Ty has ever been married. They have known one another for three years and have been living together for eight months. They seriously consider their arrangement to be a trial period and if it works out they plan to be married.

Vi does not entirely approve of the arrangement, but she does accept Susan's right to live her own life. She has met and likes Ty.

Ted totally disapproves. "If he ever shows up around here I'll go after him with the shotgun," he declares. A hard-drinking, hot-tempered, authoritarian man, it is conceivable that he would be capable of acting on his threat. He makes no secret of his antipathy toward orientals, Japanese in particular. He has not met Ty.

Susan still visits her parents periodically, but these occasions are strained and uncomfortable.

There has been no serious, open discussion of the matter.

Step 2: Define the Problem

Here it is Susan and Ty's cohabitation.

Step 3: Ideal Solutions

In this situation there are actually three different ideal solutions:

- Ted's ideal solution—Ty drops out of the picture.

- Vi's ideal solution—Ted comes to recognize that Susan has the right to do what she is doing, accepts the arrangement, and treats Susan and Ty civilly.

- Susan's ideal solution—Her parents accept the situation matter-of-factly, as Ty's parents have done. She and Ty have made a considered and mature decision about which she has no qualms. She understands that it is her parents who have the problem and need to do something about it. She is troubled by Ted's attitude toward Ty.

Ted's solution is totally incompatible with the other two and his attitude is largely responsible for the unhappiness that attends it. He does not recognize nor admit that his stubbornness and hostility are the cause of the conflict.

Step 4: Feasibility of Ideal Solution

- Ted—Getting rid of Ty is not possible. Ty and Susan may eventually break up, but any attempt to force this would backfire. Even Ted knows this.

- Vi—Reforming Ted is not likely to happen. Yet, Vi realizes that Ted is at the heart of the problem and, if matters are to improve, the effort to change his attitude has to be made.

- Susan—Though she hopes for an improved relationship with her parents (mainly Ted), she believes that it is not up to her to initiate action. Even if matters remain unchanged, it will not greatly affect her and Ty. The problem belongs with her parents and it is up to them to deal with it.

Step 5: Alternative Solutions

- Ted—None

- Vi—1. Accept matters as they are, uncomfortable as that is.
  2. Adopt Ted's view of the situation.
  3. Align herself more closely and firmly with Susan and Ty.

- Susan—Susan needs no alternatives, but she does have these options:
  1. Accept matters as they are.
  2. Discontinue seeing her parents.
  3. Break off relations with Ty.

Step 6: Sub-strategies Toward an Ideal Solution

Assuming:

1. If matters are to improve, Ted's attitudes toward Susan and Ty must change, *and*
2. This change in Ted will not occur spontaneously, and
3. Susan has no direct role to play in initiating steps toward a solution.

It is up to Vi to take action to resolve the conflict. To accomplish this, open discussion with Ted is required. *Vi recognizes at this point that she owns the problem, even though she has not authored it.* (See Chapter 4.) Vi sees that direct confrontation with Ted is called for. She is either able or unable to do this.

I. A. If she is able she will have to inform Ted directly of her concern about their relationship with Susan and her desire to discuss it fully and to work toward a better resolution of matters.

 B. If she is *unable* she must:
 B-1: Adopt one of her alternative solutions *or*
 B-2: Get help so that she becomes capable of confrontation.

If confrontation does take place, Ted will either

II. C. Agree to discuss, *or*

 D. Reject discussion. In this event Vi has the choice of:
 D-1 Dropping the matter and adopting an alternative
 D-2 Forcing discussion by introducing threats or imposing sanctions. This is a dangerous tactic because threats are often not taken seriously, are bluffs, or cannot be acted upon.

Vi's strategy to this point is sketched in Figure 6.

If Ted agrees to discussion, this can be carried out under a variety of different arrangements that Vi may propose. Possibilities include:

 C-1 She and Ted can talk it through alone.
 C-2 She, Ted, and Susan discuss (Susan and Ted willing).
 C-3 She, Ted, Susan, and Ty discuss (Susan, Ty, and Ted willing).

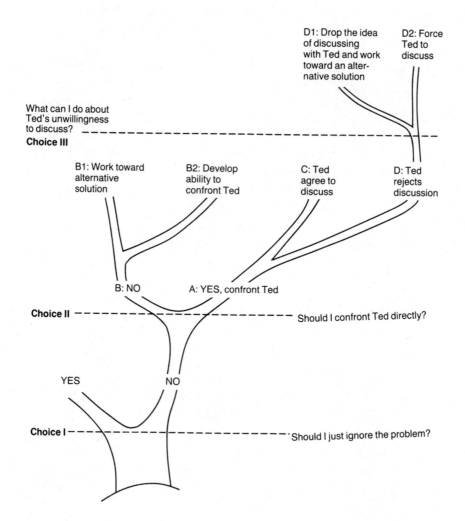

Fig. 6. Vi's substrategies toward an ideal solution in the Susan–Ty cohabitation problem.

C-4 She, Ted, and some respected and trusted third
party (friend, relative, counselor) acting as
moderator discuss.

E. Whatever the format, Ted may not participate
openly,using the occasion as a launching pad for self-
justification or denunciation of others. If that occurs, Vi
will have to:
E-1 Confront Ted, calling for open discussion.
E-2 Fall back on an alternative solution.

F. If the discussion is held openly it may either
F-1 Succeed or partly succeed in changing Ted. In this
case Vi's 'ideal' or an improved 'alternative
solution' may be attainable.
F-2 Fail or make matters worse. In this eventuality,
Vi will have to go to an alternative solution.

Figure 7 traces these remaining steps in Vi's decision-
making process.

Step 7: Consequences of Alternative Solutions

For Susan and Vi, the most tolerable 'alternative solution'
is to keep matters as they are, uncomfortable as that may be.
The other options would have destructive consequences.
Even accepting the status quo is perilous because it seems
probable that Susan and Ty will eventually marry. When that
occurs it will be a whole new ball game for everyone.

Step 8: Review

Having carried the analysis to this point, Vi would review the substrategies that she has worked out with someone
who knows the situation and is capable of bringing a fresh
and independent viewpoint to it.

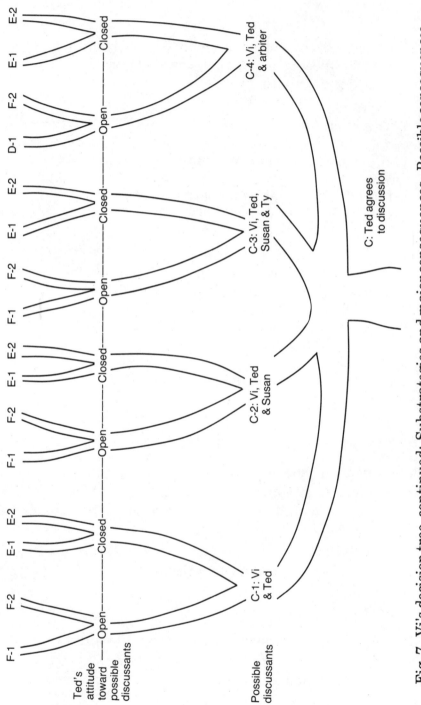

Fig. 7. Vi's decision tree, continued: Substrategies and major consequences. Possible consequences are: F-1, Strategy succeeds or partly succeeds in changing Ted; F-2, Strategy fails or makes matters worse; E-1, Confront Ted demanding open discussion; E-2, Go to alternative solution.

Step 9: Act

If the review step confirms Vi's assessment, then the time has come for her to take action in a fashion consistent with the steps she has charted out.

Step 10: Backup Strategy

In this instance, all decision points have a backup or alternative strategy written into the plan. If any of the steps to a solution were to misfire badly and actually make the situation worse than it already is, Vi must develop plans for dealing with those eventualities. Some of the developments she might have to face could include:

- Ted forbids her to have anything to do with Susan and Ty.
- Ted abuses her physically or psychologically.
- Ted walks out on her.
- Susan breaks off contact entirely.

Our example also omits certain possibilities. Ted may have devised some strategies of his own that we have not presented simply because, given his disposition and frame of mind, anything he might advocate would likely abridge the rights of the other individuals involved and would almost certainly have the effect of worsening matters.

It also does not highlight the real dread and anguish Vi will have to endure at every point. Though the procedures we have described are orderly and straightforward, they would be carried out in an atmosphere bristling with tension and hostility that might, at any point, explode. To formulate and then try out corrective measures in such a volatile situation— even when what is being rectified is well-nigh intolerable— requires a full measure of courage and determination.

The attempt to define the problem, to think about possible solutions, and to attack the matter systematically, using previously discussed ideas about the proper tactics to employ and their likely consequences, can only improve the process

that is more commonly carried out on the spur of the moment
—emotionally, angrily, punitively. Quite possibly the 'ideal
solution' (if it can even be found among all of the possible
solutions that exist) will exceed the ability of any specific individual to achieve. But the disposition to deal with a problem
and its roots dispassionately is an improvement on the usual
alternatives—lashing out blindly or suffering in silence.

Finally, a word for those who would condemn rational
efforts to solve problems by arguing that the approach strips
the essential joy—the 'human' quality—from life. That danger is about as likely as being kicked to death by butterflies—
what, after all, is more uniquely human than an attempt at
rationality, however infrequently we may succeed?

CHAPTER 19

AN EXERCISE IN
DECISION-MAKING

The work itself is fine;
it's the decisions that kill you.

Introduction

We will now present a do-it-yourself, logically sequenced series of exercises that will help you to work through the steps involved in resolving conflicts with your adult children. The exercise will set up procedures to follow when making your careful and detailed analysis, and will help you develop both the determination and the resources you need to rectify a troublesome situation.

Our aim is to help you achieve an optimal solution to the problem. But the method will be successful in accomplishing this only to the extent you are willing to spend the time and effort to analyze the dilemma thoroughly and carefully. The procedure depends entirely on your ability and willingness to be honest with yourself. At the least you should be willing to admit (if the facts point in that direction) that your problems may be imaginary, something that you have fabricated; that you may be the reason for the conflict, whatever it is; and that you, despite your real concern, may not have the legal or moral right to be involved. If you cannot acknowledge these *possibilities*, then you are simply not ready to look into the problem.

Even if you eventually realize that you yourself are in some way responsible for your plight, that does not mean that you are helpless. The procedures described here can only help you deal with the problem more effectively, more judiciously, and more comfortably. If the problem is indeed an intractable one, you are still able to change the way that it affects you. And though a situation may persist, there is no good reason to allow it to cause stress, which may entail damaging physical and psychological consequences for you. You may in fact be able to attack the problem quite directly and constructively; if you cannot, then you may nonetheless be able to learn to live with it on friendlier terms.

All of the techniques that you will use here have been discussed fully in earlier parts of this book: Chapter 3 shows how family conflicts can be harmful and mentions some of the ways in which these consequences may be avoided or minimized; Chapter 4 offers help in defining problems and tells you how you can bring yourself to the point of acting on them; Chapter 18 presents and works through the principles of making rational decisions, using what have been called "ideal procedural criteria."

Following through all of the steps we present here will not guarantee you either a perfect resolution or the total elimination of the problem, whatever it may be. But if they are carefully observed, matters ought to become far more manageable, or at least more bearable.

You can accomplish all of this single-handedly if need be, though if your spouse is also troubled by the situation, then it is far better for the two of you to work it through together. Here, now, are the steps. Remember:

- Start at the beginning!
- Be thorough—read carefully and skip nothing!
- Answer thoughtfully and carefully!
- Be honest!

Step 1: Defining the Problem

Exercise 1.   What is the situation that is troubling you? Describe that situation in the box below. Do not find fault with or judge the other individual or individuals concerned.

Examples: <u>Correct</u>: Janey drops the grandchildren off with us unexpectedly. Sometimes this is really awkward and inconvenient for us.
<u>Incorrect</u>: Janey is inconsiderate, self-centered and doesn't have any concern for us—as when she just turns up and drops the kids off to stay with us.

_____

_____

_____

The situation as   _____
you perceive or
experience it   _____

_____

_____

If you are not sure about how to describe the situation or have not decided how it affects you, a log of the type shown in Chapter 4 will help clarify these matters.

Exercise 2. Are there troubling, unfavorable, disapproving, or conflicting opinions (attitudes; feelings) about the situation as you have described it?

❑ Yes   ❑ No

If No, Stop! Your problem is, you've got no problem.

If Yes, who has the opinions and what are they?

You	Your Spouse	Your Child
_____	_____	_____
_____	_____	_____
_____	_____	_____
_____	_____	_____

Exercise 3. Have you discussed the situation openly and fully with the others concerned?

❑ Yes   ❑ No

If Yes, continue.

If No, take time now to initiate such discussion. Do not have it come up unexpectedly, without preparation, or as an unpleasant surprise to all concerned.

Exercise 4. What is the problem? (Sometimes the description of the situation prepared in response to Exercise 1 will serve as an adequate problem statement. If that will not do, write out the problem in the space below.)

The
problem
as you
perceive
or exper-
ience it

Exercise 5. As far as you can judge, is this the real problem?

   1. Does the problem really exist? Do you have indisputable evidence that it is actually happening? (Answer YES only if both conditions apply.)

       ❑ Yes   ❑ No

   2. The problem, as described, troubles me directly, or others with whom I am concerned.

       ❑ Yes   ❑ No

   3. Other aspects of my life in the family (sexual; marital; social) are generally satisfactory.

       ❑ Yes   ❑ No

Key for Exercise 5

	a	*b*	*c*	*d*	*e*	*f*	*g*	*h*
1.	Y	Y	Y	Y	N	N	N	N
2.	Y	N	Y	N	N	Y	N	Y
3.	Y	Y	N	N	N	N	Y	Y

If your answers followed pattern *a*, the real problem has probably been stated correctly.

If your answers followed patterns *b* or *g*, no problem exists. Stop!

If you answered patterns *c, d, e, f,* or *h*, be alert to the possibility that other problems exist.

Exercise 6. Who has what kind of problem?

   1. Does the problem really exist? Do you have indisputable evidence that it is actually happening? (Answer YES only if both conditions apply.)

       ❑ Yes   ❑ No

   2. Do you honestly have the legal or moral *right* to be involved in the problem? (Does it affect you directly?)

       ❑ Yes   ❑ No

3. Do you honestly have the legal or moral *responsibility* to be involved in the problem?

❑ Yes ❑ No

Key for Exercise 6

	a	b	c	d	e	f	g	h
1.	Y	Y	Y	Y	N	N	N	N
2.	Y	Y	N	N	Y	Y	N	N
3.	Y	N	Y	N	N	Y	N	Y

If your answers followed patterns *a, b,* or *c,* the problem is most likely real and shared with the child.

If your answers followed pattern *d,* the problem is most likely real. It is up to the child to deal with it and it is up to you to work through your feelings.

If your answers followed patterns *e, f, g,* or *h,* the problem is imaginary. It is up to you to clarify your perceptions and work through your feelings. See Step 11.

Exercise 7. Is there independent support for your analysis so far? (Show and discuss what you have done to this point with a confidant. Ask him or her to answer this Exercise.)

❑ Yes ❑ No

If Yes, continue.

If No, get reasons for the disagreement and review Exercises 1–6 carefully. Remember, you asked for this opinion, so don't be angry with disagreement.

Summary

At this point you should have a good idea about:

• What the problem is.
• What it grows out of.

- Whether it is real or imaginary.
- Who owns it.
- Who must deal with it.

You should also have support for the correctness of your analysis.

Step 2: Finding an Ideal Solution

Exercise 8. Review and try out self-initiated procedures, such as role-playing, visualization, and projection, as presented and discussed in Chapter 4, pp. 55 to 72.

1. Is the situation likely to clear up promptly if left alone?

❑ Yes ❑ No

2. Will the resulting state of affairs, if matters are left alone, be acceptable to all concerned?

❑ Yes ❑ No

Key for Exercise 6

	a	b	c	d
1.	Y	Y	N	N
2.	Y	N	Y	N

If pattern *a*, Stop! Relax. Let things improve on their own.

If pattern *b*, *c*, or *d*, continue.

Exercise 9. Are you confident that you can take action to bring about change, especially if the action is likely to result in conflict or disagreement?

❑ Yes ❑ No

If No, carry out further self-initiated procedures or secure outside help so that the capability is acquired. *See also* Step 11.

If Yes, continue.

Exercise 10. What is your ideal solution? (Write out your version of the best, most agreeable solution for *you*.)

Your
statement_____
of the
ideal   _____
solution

Step 3: Deciding on the Feasibility of the Ideal Solution

Exercise 11. In your judgment can all individuals involved accept or live with your ideal solution comfortably?

❑ Yes   ❑ No

If Yes, continue.

If No, move to Step 4.

Exercise 12. Can the ideal solution be reached without violating any rights or freedoms of any individuals concerned?

❑ Yes   ❑ No

If Yes, continue.

If No, move to Step 4.

Exercise 13. Is the ideal solution clearly within legal or moral limits?

❑ Yes   ❑ No

If Yes, continue.

If No, move to Step 4.

Exercise 14. To achieve the ideal solution will you have to run unacceptably high risks of negative or damaging consequences?

❑ Yes   ❑ No

If Yes, move to Step 4
If No, you have a feasible solution. Move to Step 5

Step 4: Setting up Alternative Solutions

Exercise 15. In the spaces below list the advantages and disadvantages of every solution you can name. Take time to ponder this exercise carefully and to develop a complete list. Begin with the "Do nothing" alternative which is supplied. Use additional sheets of paper if necessary.

Alternative	Advantages	Disadvantages
1. Do nothing	_____	_____
2.	_____	_____
3.	_____	_____
4.	_____	_____
5.	_____	_____
6.	_____	_____
7.	_____	_____
8.	_____	_____
9.	_____	_____
10.	_____	_____

Considering the advantages and disadvantages of each alternative, decide which is the most favorable or least unfavorable). Write its number here. _____

Exercise 16. In your judgment, can all the individuals involved accept or live with the alternative solution?

   ❏ Yes   ❏ No

If Yes, continue.

If No, go to another alternative solution and return to Exercise 16.

Exercise 17. Can the alternative solution be achieved without violating any rights or freedoms of any individuals concerned?

   ❏ Yes   ❏ No

If Yes, continue.

If No, go to another alternative solution and return to Exercise 16.

Exercise 18. Is the alternative solution attainable within legal or moral limits?

   ❏ Yes   ❏ No

If Yes, continue.

If No, go to another alternative solution and return to Exercise 16.

Exercise 19. To achieve the alternative solution will you have to run unaceptably high risks of negative or damaging consequences?

   ❏ Yes   ❏ No

If Yes, go to another alternative solution and return to Exercise 16.

If No, move to STEP 5.

Repeat Exercises 16–19 with different alternative solutions until an acceptable one is found. If there is no acceptable solution then you will have to find a way to live with the problem more comfortably. In this event, go to Step 11.

Step 5: Developing Strategies Leading to an Ideal or the Best Alternative Solution

Exercise 20. List below all the strategies you can think of to get to the solution. You may be helped in this task if you remember that strategies can either take effect immediately or later on (deferred) and can be put into effect either by you acting alone (unilaterally) or, preferably, by you and all others working in concert (bilaterally.)

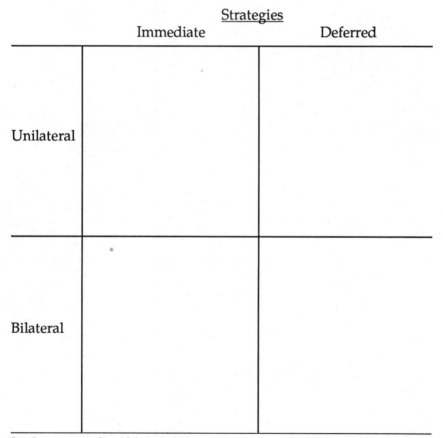

| | Strategies | |
	Immediate	Deferred
Unilateral		
Bilateral		

In the event of problems that are imaginary *(see Exercise 5)* you will need to select strategies that will help you clarify your perceptions and work through your own feelings. *(See also* Step 11.)

Step 6: Analyzing Consequences of Strategies

Exercise 21. Take each of the strategies listed in Exercise 20 and
record the consequences (positive and negative)
each will likely have for you and any others involved in the problem. (Answer completely and
thoughtfully.)

Strategy	Plusses	Minuses

Use additional sheets of paper if needed

Step 7: Making a Tentative Decision

Exercise 22. Review the strategies and their consequences. Which one looks best for all concerned?

_____

This is your tentative decision.

Exercise 23. Will you need to develop any substrategies to carry out your decision?

❑ Yes   ❑ No

If No, continue.

If Yes, list, in order, the substrategies you will need to carry out. (*See* Chapter 18, pp. 205 to 232 for discussion of this point.

1. _____

2. _____

3. _____

4. _____

5. _____

Step 8: Reviewing the Tentative Decision

Exercise 24. Repeat Steps 5, 6, and 7.

Does the Tentative Decision (Step 7) still seem best?

❑ Yes   ❑ No

If Yes, continue.

If No, select another tentative decision and repeat.

Exercise 25. Have a friend or confidant review your tentative decision. Does the reviewer agree with your decision?

❑ Yes   ❑ No

If Yes, continue.

If No, determine the reason for the disagreement and, if necessary, revise the decision and review.

Summary

At this point you will have

- Figured out the best solution possible.
- Developed various strategies to get to that solution.
- Estimated the consequences of the strategies.
- Made a tentative decision.

You should also have independent support for the soundness of that decision.

Step 9: Taking Action

Exercise 26. Take the action or actions spelled out in Step 7. Once the decision is made, act on it without undue delay.

Step 10: Readying a Backup

Exercise 27. The decision may prove to be wrong or the strategies to effect it may fail. If either of these possibilities occurs, what will be your response?

_____

_____

_____

_____

(Suggestion: Rework Steps 3–9. Under conditions of failure the problem will be changed and, in all likelihood, made worse.)

Step 11: Dealing with Insoluble or Imaginary Problems

If the problem seems to have no solution or you cannot seem to bring yourself to act on it, in your own self interest you should take whatever actions you can to minimize its effects on you.

Review Chapter 3 to get suggestions about self-help exercises that will reduce stress or conflict, and Chapter 4 to suggest ways of motivating yourself to act.

Exercise 28. Are you willing and able to seriously initiate self-help exercises in stress reduction?

❏ Yes ❏ No

If Yes, select and faithfully carry out an appropriate program of self-help. (You may also want to consider Exercise 29.)

Exercise 29. Are you willing and able to secure outside help which may enable you to combat the effects of tension and stress?

❏ Yes ❏ No

If Yes, turn to suggestions contained in Chapter 20 on getting outside help.

If Yes to Exercise 28, No to Exercise 29, return to Exercise 28.

If No to both Exercise 28 and Exercise 29, you are not doing anything about the problem or its consequences for you.

If the problem is an outgrowth of your own imagination, or exists but is none of your affair (*see* Exercise 6) you might benefit greatly from outside help which will enable you to perceive the situation differently.

Exercise 30. Are you willing to seek outside help to clarify the situation and your place and role in it?

❏ Yes ❏ No

If Yes, turn to suggestions contained in Chapter 20.

If No, you are simply allowing the situation to drag on.

SUMMARY

At this point you will have:

- Decided to act, and
- Prepared a backup strategy in case of failure, or,
- Dealt with an insoluble or imaginary problem by changing the way you perceive and respond to it, either through imposing self-help measures or by getting outside assistance.

If you have come all this way through the exercises and have not yet succeeded in moving toward a solution of the problem—or your own part in it—it may benefit you to read Chapter 3 again, carefully, prior to repeating these Steps and *Exercises* one more time.

CHAPTER 20

FINDING THE RIGHT KIND OF HELP

Introduction

Looking for help with a family conflict is not something people do every day. When this lack of experience is combined with the intense pressures such problems usually entail, and swift action is forced, the resulting choice of outside aid can prove disastrous. We will here outline procedures that will enable you to decide whether you need outside help, show you how to generate a roster of potential sources of such help and how then to narrow it down, explain what tactics you will find especially useful in securing that aid, and finally, provide you detailed listings of the major sources of both general assistance and of specific problem-oriented help. If you are guided by the procedures we recommend, you will no doubt greatly reduce the risk of wasting time and money on unqualified and/or worthless helping resources.

To find the right kind of aid, it is absolutely essential that you closely follow the suggestions, carrying out whatever search is necessary. Since chances are good that the problem has been bedeviling you for a while, a few additional days' delay ought not make that much difference. Proceed carefully, seek advice, do the research, and ask the pointed questions that need to be asked before settling on a choice.

This set of guidelines is designed for middle-aged parents in conflict with adult children. Though these conflicts are painful and troubling, they are not usually associated with severe, chronic, or disabling mental health problems. The latter require medical treatment prior to, and often simultaneously with, provision of the kind of psychological counseling or assistance that lies at the core of the recommendations here.

A Word About Conflict

Conflict usually signifies the presence of disagreement and strife between individuals or groups, and many family troubles fit that definition neatly.

For psychologists, conflict also refers to a process that goes on entirely within the individual. Its end result is the vacillation or uncertainty that occurs when an individual experiences competing tendencies to approach and avoid some objective or goal. The individual who has an appointment for an important job interview on the eighty-eighth floor of the Empire State building, and who also has a deathly fear of elevators, suffers such a conflict. So, too does the middle-aged parent who is acutely concerned about an adult child's behavior (something the child is thought to be doing or not doing), but is loath to say something about it to the child.

Conflict also occurs when a problem exists, but one is prevented from dealing with it. Being unable to take measures to resolve a difficulty almost inevitably leads to distress and the feeling of helplessness that is commonplace in the relationship between parents and children.

Resources do exist to help individuals manage such feelings when their owners cannot handle them unaided. If the underlying situation or the feelings it engenders can be dealt with unaided by the parent, well and good. If it cannot (or if it is something that the parent has fabricated or dreamed up), outside assistance may well be required.

Deciding When Outside Help Is Needed

You yourself must decide when you need outside help. Deciding to seek help means that you have concluded such assistance will either enable you to deal with a problem more effectively or, alternatively, will make it possible for you to ride it through comfortably or observe it more objectively. When you have an unresolved problem with a child (and here we assume that you have already discussed the situation openly with the child and other persons involved), you have the first hint that help might be useful.

"Needing" help is one thing; whether or not one will actually look for it is something else. The major bar that people confront to securing or using help, however necessary such help may be, is the conviction that one ought not require it and that one is in some way better off for not asking for or having to rely on external assistance. If it makes sense to flounder, to wallow in feelings of inadequacy, frustration, doubt, or anxiety, then it makes sense to do it "your way." Though it may be a sign of strength or "character" to shun aid, this attitude simply encourages to let our problems drag on, become ingrained, and grow more susceptible to bad solutions. So, if you are experiencing a family problem that

- You don't know what to do about
- Causes you feelings of distress, anxiety, frustration, anger, helplessness
- You can't seem to get around to tackling
- Seems to be one that only you recognize or take seriously

it may be time for you to think seriously about getting outside help.

Tactics for Looking for
and Getting Outside Help

Once you have made the decision to look for help, there are several steps you can take that will point you to the right source. These steps are:

1. Define your problem.
2. Build a list of potential sources of help.
3. Canvass these sources to determine what fees, qualifications, conditions, or requirements may be entailed.
4. Make a tentative choice.
5. Review your choice with a confidant.
6. Make a final selection.

Defining the Problem

The kind of help you finally settle on should be determined by the problem that has brought you to the realization that you need assistance. If you are unable to deal with the fact that your daughter is living with someone, taking the problem to Al-Anon won't do you much good—unless she is also an alcoholic, chances are they will not even want you around. Actually, this decision should not be difficult because you have reached a point where you recognize the existence of a problem for which you need outside help. State this problem. Preferably write it out briefly. Here are a few examples of problem statements.

> Our son is an alcoholic who neglects and abuses his wife and children. This distresses me terribly.

> I am continually angry with and getting to the point where I can hardly talk to our son who doesn't work and simply hangs out with us at home. I want to be able to discuss it with him sanely and productively.

Our daughter has always been something of a flittertigibbet, especially when it comes to choosing friends and in her personal relationships. I worry all of the time that she's going to get into serious trouble. I would like to be able to have more confidence in her.

I am driven to distraction by the constant arguments between my husband and son. I'm afraid to say or do anything about the situation. Yet, it is tearing me apart.

Our son has openly declared that he is a homosexual. I am so upset by this and by what our relatives and friends will think that I just don't know what to do or how to handle it.

Now, take a look at what you've written. The statement will nearly always contain some key words or phrases that reveal the condition you are trying to correct or find relief from—"...alcoholic...distresses," "...angry...can hardly talk to our son," "...worry...would like to have more confidence," and so on. These key words will focus your search for the right kind of assistance.

Building a List of Potential Help Sources

The business of providing help for troubled individuals is a growth industry in this country. There is no scarcity of assistance; as a matter of fact, there are so many varieties of help available that selecting the most suitable and appropriate resource may be quite difficult and confusing. To help you thread your way through this almost impenetrable maze, we have named the principal locations in which information on the major helping resources is likely to be found. In approaching any one of these resources, you need always to keep the nature of your problem firmly in mind. Failing to do so will inevitably leave you wading through a great swamp of irrelevant information. In fact, that will probably happen to some degree no matter how careful you are. Here, then, are the suggested starting points.

*The annotated list of help sources that appears later in this
chapter.* It names and comments on the general kinds
of assistance available and also provides the names of
organizations and services that will deal with your
specific problems—unemployment, unwanted pregnancies, and so on. All organizations named in it will
be found in the white pages of most telephone books.

A friend or adviser. You should always inquire of individuals who, through their positions in life or from
their personal experience, are able to offer useful suggestions. A friend who has obtained help for his or her
own similar problem will generally be able to offer
knowledgeable advice. Your lawyer, doctor, clergyman, or a relative will often be able to do likewise.

The Yellow Pages of the telephone directory. Your phone
book will list specialized sources of help, providing the
names of individuals or agencies that concern themselves with each of the problem areas set forth below.
You then need to select those that bear most directly on
your situation and place your calls.

Alcoholism Information and Treatment Centers	Includes names of public and private referral, detoxification, and other facilities available for the treatment of alcoholics or their families
Birth Control Information Centers	Gives clinic, hotline, planned parenthood, and other numbers
Crisis Intervention Services	Will commonly list places to call for emergencies involving alcohol, drugs, various kinds of abuse, and suicide
Drug Abuse (Addiction) Information and Treatment centers	Lists facilities available for treatment of individuals using substances, or for the family affected by this abuse.

(continued)

Drug Abuse (Addiction) Information and Treatment centers (*continued*)	Includes names of public or private treatment centers, detoxification programs, and other resources available to drug users or their families. In some places a special effort is being made to identify and treat older people using dangerous drugs to excess.
Emergency Medical and Surgical Services	Will include names of medically oriented Mental Health emergency services.
Family Planning Information Centers	Largely duplicates Birth Control Information Centers listings
Human Services Organizations	Organizations providing assistance to various categories of individuals or groups. Will name groups concerned about welfare of children, prisoners, some ethnic minorities, and so on.
Marriage and Family Counselors	Trained and licensed individuals who offer marital and family assistance for a fee
Mental Health Services	Names of organizations providing referral to or direct mental health treatment services
Mental Retardation and Developmentally Disabled Services	Names of organizations or groups concerned with or offering services for individuals so categorized or for their families
Parents Guidance Instruction	Largely duplicates Marriage and Family Counselors entry
Physicians, Psychiatrists, Psychoanalysts	Medical doctors specializing in the treatment of individuals with chronic and more serious psychological problems

(*continued*)

Psychologists
(*continued*)

Psychologists in private practice who meet educational and licensing requirements. Individual entries will usually state the highest degree earned and the kinds of problems specialized in, such as individual therapy, family difficulties, couples, women, Gestalt, biofeedback, behavioral, stress and pain management, etc. There may be a Psychologist Information Bureau also listed which can help direct you to the resource most relevant to your problem

Rehabilitation
Services

Lists agencies and groups helping in the rehabilitation of persons with a wide range of physical, psychological, or social problems

Schools, Universities
and Colleges (Academic)

Sometimes the telephone company errs in this entry by including non-academic institutions, such as modeling colleges and other places that carry the name "college" in their title. If in doubt, check the *College Blue Book* for the names of accredited institutions of higher learning. Your local library can also help here.

Social Service and
Welfare Organizations

Public and private organizations that exist to help individuals in trouble. Both treatment and referral facilities will be found under this heading

Social Workers

Trained and licensed social workers who help individuals with personal or family problems

By making contact with each of the service providers relevant to the problem you confront, you will generally come up with a raft of suggestions. There are additional references you might locate and consult, although they are not likely to add much at this point. In the interest of completeness, however, these backup resources include:

Local-Level Resources

Family Service Agency. Usually maintains a list of all sources of help available to families with problems and offers direct assistance with many of them.

Community Planning Council (Community Welfare Council or Agency). In many localities this is an organization that plans and coordinates programs designed to help individuals and groups in the community. It will often publish a directory of such community-based services.

City or County Government. Local governments usually support and maintain a variety of programs, the nature and location of which can be determined by calling the general information number provided.

The Library (Community, regional, or college or university). Libraries everywhere have trained staff who can help you find information. They also collect and file documents that might be relevant to your problem.

Community Switchboard. Some communities maintain a "hot-line" service intended to put individuals in touch with local help resources.

Consumer Groups. A few communities are fortunate enough to have consumer groups that have collected and published directories of individuals engaged in treatment. These often list their specialties, fees, and other pertinent information. Your local Mental Health Society ought to know whether such information is available in your area.

State Level Resources

The State Department of Health will maintain lists of state-supported facilities or programs. Such lists can be secured by writing or calling the state capital, by writing your elected state representative, or by calling the local branch of the State Health Department if there is one in your community.

The State Department of Licensing (Bureau of Occupational and Vocational Standards, Board of Examiners, etc.) maintains lists of individuals licensed to offer services to the public. Included in such occupations would be physicians, psychologists, social workers, and other counseling specialties. Write or call for list.

Statewide Associations of Professional Groups (Counselors, Psychologists, Social Workers) list individuals who are members in good standing of such professional societies. Addresses available from the local library; usually such groups will bear such names as "New York State Psychological Association," etc.

Federal or National Level Resources

National Institute of Mental Health of the US Department of Health and Human Services has a directory of federally funded Community Mental Health Centers. Facilities are listed alphabetically by name so that locating those in your community may take some digging. A directory can be secured from your local HHS office or by writing NIMH, 5600 Fishers Lane, Rockville, MD 20857.

Toll-Free Numbers. Listed below are a few toll-free telephone numbers from which information and advice on the type of problem indicated can often be obtained.

Acquired Immune Deficiency Syndrome (AIDS)
    National Gay/Lesbian Crisis Line   800-221-7044

Child Abuse
    Parents Anonymous Hotline   800-532-0386
    Child Help USA   800-422-4453

Down's Syndrome
    National Down's Syndrome Society Hotline 800-221-4602

Drug Abuse
    National Cocaine Hotline   800-262-2463
    National Institute on Drug Abuse   800-638-2045

Handicaps
    Crisis Line for the Handicapped   800-426-4263

Independent Living
    Lifeline Systems   800-451-0525

Pregnancy
    National Abortion Federation   800-638-6725

As you go along, list the names and telephone numbers of individuals or agencies that seem to hold promise of providing you help. Once you have compiled such a list—and you can save you much time if you keep it to ten possibilities or so—you are in a position to proceed with inquiries about your specific problem.

Canvassing Your List of Possible Help Sources

Use the telephone to get in touch with those sources of help that seem most relevant to your problem. In calling, tell the person who answers the phone that you have a problem you need help with. Be ready to describe the problem briefly, if asked. Go on to inform the other person that you'd like information about the services their group is offering. Some of the questions you may wish to ask might include:

- Does the source deal with my kind of problem?
- Is there a waiting period? How long?

- How often must I come in?
- Will this be an individual or group experience?
- What are the fees?
- What are the qualifications of the individual offering the assistance? Educational background? Previous experience? Licensed or certificated?
- What methods or procedures are likely to be followed? A wide variety of approaches is used in individual or group counseling or therapy. Some of the names of these are Gestalt, Behavioral, Transactional Analysis, Rogerian, Directive, Eclectic, Conjoint, and Multiple. If you are unfamiliar with these different approaches, how precisely they proceed, and what outlay of time, effort, and expense they may demand of you, ask for details and clarification.

All of this information has to do with the kind and quality of help that you will receive. But in addition to keeping a record of the answers, you should jot down your impression of the way in which your inquiry was handled. Were you treated politely, considerately, with interest and concern, or were you given abrupt, off-handed replies? This information should also be taken into account in making a final choice—after all, the amount of progress you will make toward resolving the problem depends in part on how you feel about the specific approach being employed. If you are favorably impressed, optimistic, and positive, you will very likely do better than in other, less agreeable circumstances.

Making a Tentative Choice

With the canvassing done, you have reached the point at which a tentative choice about where to go for help can be made. How urgently you need help and the dollar amount you are prepared pay for it are important considerations. Remember, however, that most health insurance plans or health maintenance programs will defray at least part of the costs; investigate that possibility carefully. The qualifications of the person who will assist you is another important and somewhat tricky issue. In general, you should restrict your choice to:

1. Someone who has at least the equivalent of a Master's Degree in a relevant subject (psychology, sociology, social work) from a reputable institution of higher learning. Names of accredited schools and their programs are listed in the *College Blue Book,* which will be on the reference shelf of almost any library, or
2. Someone who has a license or certificate issued by the state that permits him or her to practice as a counselor, social worker, or psychologist. (State licensing boards usually make the Master's degree the minimum educational qualification.) *and*
3. Someone who has had significant experience or background in the field.

Though these precautions may seem excessive, the fact is that the human services field has always attracted more than its share of charlatans and quacks ready to take advantage of the vulnerability of unhappy, beleaguered people. The woods are full of palm or card readers, psychics, mystics, astrologers, and a bewildering assortment of others who stand ready to help you with your problem—any problem— for a fee. When you entrust yourself and your family to any type of counselor, you are literally putting yourselves in his or her hands. You owe it to yourself and your family to seek out the best, most warmly recommended, most skilled advisor whose services you can command.

With respect to the methods or procedures to be used, all of the techniques regularly employed have enjoyed their successes and failures. Success seems to depend to some degree upon the individual practitioner chosen, and to some degree upon the characteristics of the individual seeking help, so that a prescription for success here is just not possible. Middle-aged people probably find it rather more difficult to function openly in group settings than do their younger counterparts. Thus if you have any qualms about making public disclosures, or engaging in public confrontation, you may be more comfortable in an individual, one-on-one counseling situation. However, my experience has demonstrated again and again that some of the most powerful and effective techniques of mediating change are most commonly experienced in groups. Thus the potential advantages of participating in a group experience may well outweigh any prospective disadvantages or discomforts.

Checking Your Decision With a Confidant

Here's that trusted friend again. Tell this individual your problem, your decision to seek help, the places you've looked into, and what you are now proposing to do. Let him or her review these efforts with you, and solicit comments, suggestions, or criticisms about your decision and the steps you took to reach it. If he or she agrees with what you've done, and with what you propose to do, fine. If not, review the plan again and make any adjustments that seem called for.

Choosing Your Help Source

This is the easy part. Call up the person or the organization you have decided to use and set up your first appointment.

Sources of Help—An Annotated List

In America today you can readily find a competent advisor to help you with just about any type of problem you might suffer. In the following material, I provide an annotated list of the major resources likely to prove helpful in solving the family conflicts with which this book is concerned, a list that will help you to decide where best to look for help.

In considering sources of help, you should remember that we have incorporated a "Getting Help" section in the discussion of each of the specific problems treated in Parts 3 and 4. Be sure to review that material, as well as what is presented below, when developing your plans for enlisting aid.

To make the information as useful and accessible as possible, it has been broken into four lists. The first of these provides specific information on the traditional, general assistance obtainable in most communities, either from individuals or public agencies. The second covers help that may be available through community-based private agencies, institutions, or groups. Treatment in these settings may take a variety of forms and may occur in a number of different contexts.

The third section deals with specific problems that individuals may need help with—from alcohol, drugs, and the like to stress reduction. The resources named here may include "nontraditional" ones, that is, they may not involve trained professionals. However, they will employ individuals who have had first-hand experience with the problem being addressed. This sort of peer self-help can be especially effective in bringing individuals to the point at which they can address, reconceptualize, and resolve problems. The final section offers suggestions about where to go in a crisis when immediate help is essential.

Traditional General Help Sources

Traditional help usually entails aiding the individual, family, or group in a counseling-type of setting in which a professionally trained person will be present and will assume responsibility for the nature and direction of the treatment. Such help can be secured in either private or public settings. Almost any individual or family problem can be taken to such a place initially; referrals to more specialized resources may follow.

Private Settings

Private Helping Sources

Helper	Where found	Fees[1,2,3]	Waiting period?
Marriage & family counselor	Phone book, yellow pgs.	$60-90/hr	No
Psychiatrist	Phone book, yellow pgs.	$125+/hr	No
Psychologist	Phone book, yellow pgs.	$65-100/hr	No
Social Worker	Phone book, yellow pgs.	$60-90/hr	No

[1]Figures given are ranges for a middle-sized western city. Will run higher in large metropolitan centers, less in smaller places.

[2]Many individual therapists will adjust their fees according to the ability of the individual to pay; those just starting a practice will often change less than established practitioners.

[3]Costs for group sessions run less, ordinarily one-third to one-half of the individual fee.

Public Settings

Public services will ordinarily be provided by one or another of the kinds of professionals listed above, usually in a clinic setting. Such services are commonly subsidized in part by governmental or charitable contributions.

Public Helping Sources

Name	Where found	Fees*	Waiting period	Comment
(Community) Mental Health Clinic	Phone book white pgs.	Sliding scale	1,2	Provides extensive kinds and modes of treatment

(continued)

Public Health Sources *(continued)*

Name	Where found	Fees*	Waiting period	Comment
Community College	Phone book white pgs.	Sliding scale	3	
College or University Public Clinic	Phone book yellow pgs.	Sliding scale	3	Services may be provided by advanced students under faculty supervision
Dept. of Social Welfare/Services	Phone book governmental listings	None	None	Primarily for referrals
Family Service Agency	Phone book white pgs.	Sliding scale	1,2	Deals with large variety of problems; excellent starting point
Mental Health Association	Phone book white pgs.	—	—	Referral source
Neighborhood Program	Phone book yellow pgs.	Sliding scale	1,2	May target ethnic minorities, poor
Veteran's Administration	Phone book governmental listings	None	2	For eligible veterans

[1]Emergency consultations usually available.
[2]Short waiting period (1-2 weeks) may be required.
[3]Longer waiting period; some times when services unavailable.
*Where a sliding scale of fees applies, charges usually are determined by ability to pay and no one is refused treatment for lack of funds.

Help Available Through Private Institutions, Agencies, or Groups

In some of the groups named below, aid may be provided by individuals who do not have the usual academic credentials. However, this lack of formal training will be offset by substantial experience and familiarity with the problems being presented.

Private Institutions

Type of group	Where found	Fees*	Waiting period	Comment
Employer	Place of work	None	None	Many larger private or public employers support programs designed to help employees or their families
Ethnic	Phone book white or yellow pages	Usually none	Varies	All ethnic programs are designed to respond to the special problems and needs of minority group members
Asian	"	"	"	
Chinese	"	"	"	
Filipino	"	"	"	
Japanese	"	"	"	
Indochinese	"	"	"	
Black	"	"	"	
NAACP	"	"	"	
Urban League	"	"	"	
Hispanic	"	"	"	
Latino	"	"	"	
La Raza	"	"	"	
Mexican-American	"	"	"	
Puerto Rican	"	"	"	
Indian	"	"	"	
Native American	"	"	"	
Inter-Tribal Council	"	"	"	

(continued)

Private Institutions *(continued)*

Type of group	Where found	Fees*	Waiting period	Comment
Pastoral–Religious				
Catholic Social Services	Phone book white pgs.	Sliding scale	Varies	Wide variety of services available to all
Jewish Federation	"	None	"	Membership sometimes required
Protestant denominations: Lutheran Methodist Presbyterian Episcopal Salvation Army etc.	"	Varies	"	Character, extent and type of services will vary greatly, from full professional clinical facilities to less extensive and more specialized forms of aid. Other religious groups may be involved depending on local availability
YMCA YWCA	"	Varies with the service provided	"	Provides a range of services, groups, clinics, and other types of help directed at families or individuals
Women				
Women's Center	"	Varies	"	Provides a variety of resources and help for women
National Orgn. for Women	"	—	—	Primarily a referral source

Sources of Help with Specific Problems

Problem and helping source	Location of helping source	Comment
Abuse (spousal or child)	Phone book white pgs	
Social Welfare Dept. Adult or Child Protective Services Family Service Agency Local Law Enforcement (Police/Sheriff)		
Parents Anonymous		To aid parents wanting to avoid abusing children
Women's Center NOW		Referral source
Alcohol Abuse	Phone book yellow pgs.	
AA AL-ANON		All AA programs subscribe to the underlying philosophy of the
ALATEEN Alcoholism Council (local) Alcoholism programs Ethnic Alcoholism programs		organization Best initial referral source
Employer		Where offered, employer programs to counter alcoholism have been quite effective
Health Maintenance Organization Salvation Army Dept. of Social Welfare		
Volunteers of America		Emphasis is on helping the public inebriate

(continued)

Sources of Help with Specific Problems *(continued)*

Problem and helping source	Location of helping source	Comment
Drug abuse		
(Local) Drug Council	Phone book yellow pgs.	Primarily a referral source. Likely to maintain a "hotline"
(Local) Treatment Centers		
AA		Sponsors some drug therapy
Alcoholism Council	Phone book white pgs.	Makes referrals on drug problems and queries
Employment/Job Placement/Vocational Counseling		
Community College Placement Bureau	Phone book white pages	For eligible individuals. May offer testing and search strategies as well as referrals
College or University Placement Bureau	"	"
Employment Agencies	Phone book yellow pages	Act primarily as job brokers although some offer "aptitude" and other forms of testing. Fee charging. Have some unscrupulous operators who conspire with employers to bilk applicants. Check first with the Better Business Bureau or the Dept. of Consumer Affairs
(State) Employment Development Dept.	Phone book governmental listings	Do some limited aptitude and interest testing and make referrals of applicants to jobs. Also provide counseling.

(continued)

Sources of Help with Specific Problems *(continued)*

Problem and helping source	Location of helping source	Comment
Employment, Job Placement, Vocational Counseling (cont'd)		
NAACP	Phone book white pages	In some localities òffers job training programs. Referral source
Social Welfare-Employment	Phone book governmental listings	Aids individuals with potential for employment, education, or training to find and utilize community resources
Urban League	Phone book white pages	Provides counseling, work experience, on-the-job training opportunities for eligible persons
Vocational Consultants	Phone book white pages	Private individuals furnishing various kinds of assistance in the job search including resume preparation. Check with Better Business Bureau
Women's Center	Phone book white pages	Help women define and seek out employment goals. Referral source
Financial/Money Management		
Bank or Financial Institution	Phone book white pages	
Consumer Credit Counseling Service	Phone book white pages	Provide counseling and help on a wide variety of money management problems. Excellent and disinterested resource
Employer	At work	Where available, useful help source

(continued)

Sources of Help with Specific Problems *(continued)*

Problem and helping source	Location of helping source	Comment
Gambling		
Gamblers Anonymous	Phone book white pages	A self-help group for compulsive gamblers run along the lines of and with many of AA's assumptions
Gam-Anon	"	A self-help group for families of gamblers much like AL-ANON in operation and intent
Handicaps/Disabilities		
Center for Independent Living	"	Provides a wide variety of services aimed at helping the seriously disabled achieve occupational, fiscal, and personal independence
Family Service Agency	"	Provides many help resources and makes referrals to appropriate agencies
Support group for (name of disease or condition)	Community Services Directory	
Homosexuality		
Gay Alliance	Phone book yellow pgs.	Referral source
Support group for parents of gay/lesbian children	Phone book white pgs. or through Gay Student Association at a local college	

(continued)

Sources of Help with Specific Problems *(continued)*

Problem and helping source	Location of helping source	Comment
Individual and Family Development/ Mental Health Services	Phone book yellow pgs. (Psychologists, Social Workers, Human Services, family counselors, etc.)	Read directory entries to identify individuals or groups specializing in or offering the sorts of services needed
College or University Counseling Center or Clinic	Phone book white pgs.	Will know of and be able to direct callers to appropriate sources in the community; often offer such services to the public on campus
Women's Center	Phone book white pgs.	Should be aware of facilities especially designed for women. May offer such programs directly
YMCA/YWCA	"	The "Ys" often make these kinds of services a part of their programs
Legal		
Attorneys	Phone book yellow pgs.	Select an attorney (if you need and can afford one) in the same way you would get other kinds of help. See steps at the beginning of this chapter
Legal Aid Society	Phone book white pgs.	Furnishes free legal services in civil matters—domestic relations, unemployment, etc.—to eligible low income clients

(continued)

Sources of Help with Specific Problems *(continued)*

Problem and helping source	Location of helping source	Comment
Legal (cont'd.)		
Family Court Services	Phone book governmental listings	Where available, provides a variety of services having to do with marriage, child custody, dissolution of marriage
Public Defender	Phone book white pgs.	Argues the legal defense of persons charged with a crime. Eligibility based on income
Referral Service	Phone book white pgs. (under local Bar Assn.)	A referral service supplied by some local bar associations. Directs callers to appropriate legal help sources after consultation. Small fee may be required
Pregnancy/Abortion/Family Planning		
Catholic Social Services	Phone book white pgs.	Offers pre-marriage and marriage counseling, family planning programs, etc.
Planned Parenthood	"	Provides diversified information and services for all, including birth control counseling, education, pregnancy termination and sterilization. Low fees
Pregnancy Consultation Center	"	A "right-to-life" group that counsels persons about alternatives to abortion
Social Welfare- Family Planning	Phone book governmental listings	Gives, on request, information (counseling) on family planning. Refers clients to other available aid and

(continued)

Sources of Help with Specific Problems *(continued)*

Problem and helping source	Location of helping source	Comment
Pregnancy/Abortion/Family Planning (cont'd.)		
Social Welfare Family Planning		helping resources of the community
Women's Center	Phone book white pgs.	Can provide counseling, information, referrals
Stress Management		
Psychologists, Social Workers	Phone book yellow pgs.	Look for individuals who offer stress-reducing techniques like behavioral treatment, biofeedback, meditation, relaxation, yoga, etc
Acupuncture, biofeedback, meditation instruction, yoga	Phone book yellow pages	Practitioners listed under those headings. Since there may be no bars to practice these specialties, check credentials first through Consumer Affairs, Better Business Bureau, etc.

Help With Crises

When a sudden, serious emergency erupts, its very unexpectedness and the need to do something immediately tends to impel hasty and, all too often, ill-considered action.

Before tackling such a crisis, it is best to try consultation. If, at the least, you can discover what your options are, your decisions will almost certainly be sounder. Most communities maintain a 24-hour service that refers callers to organizations offering assistance on a wide range or problems, and provides their telephone numbers. The name of this service will vary from place to place—Community Switchboard, Talk

Line, Hot Line, Crisis Intervention, and so on. The emergency listings in the first section of your telephone directory will usually name this resource. In addition, local law enforcement officials will provide assistance with any of the emergencies listed below.

Crisis Help Resources

Crisis	Help resource
Alcohol	(Community) Alcohol Detoxification Center
Beating or assault (wife or children)	(Community) Women's Center
Drug	(Community) Drug Detoxification Center
Psychiatric	(Hospital) Psychiatric Emergency Services
Rape	(Community) Rape Crisis Center
Suicide	(Community) Suicide Prevention Center

Fortunately, the serious emergencies we have been discussing crop up in only a very few families. The majority of the problems treated in this book, distressing though they are, plainly do not qualify as crises. For all of them there is the latitude to search out alternatives, to move deliberately and thoughtfully, and to make optimal use of the procedures and rosters of available helping resources described in *Coping with Your Grown Children*. In short, I am confident that you—the loving, but troubled and perplexed parent—now enjoy an excellent grounding in how best to make informed, rational decisions about nearly every imaginable type of problem you and your mature children may confront in your continuing lives together.

Index